# NO SWEAT FITNESS

◇

## THE EVERYDAY GUIDE TO HEALTHY LIVING FOR THE '90s

## TANIA ALEXANDER

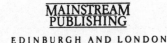

MAINSTREAM
PUBLISHING

EDINBURGH AND LONDON

First published in Great Britain 1992 by
MAINSTREAM PUBLISHING COMPANY (EDINBURGH) LTD
7 Albany Street
Edinburgh EH1 3UG

ISBN 1 85158 476 5 (paper)

A catalogue record for this book is available from the British Library

Book design by James Hutcheson
Illustrations by Irene Barry

Filmset in Monotype Garamond by Selwood Systems, Midsomer Norton
Printed and Bound in Great Britain by Billings & Sons Ltd, Worcester

Although every exercise in this book has been devised with safety in mind, exercise should always be approached with care and caution. The exercises detailed in this book assume that you are in good health. The safety guidelines in this book should be carefully followed and if you are in any doubt about your suitability to do any of the exercises, please approach your doctor first. The publishers and author cannot accept responsibility for any injury or damage suffered as a result of attempting an exercise in this book.

To my darling husband, Stuart

# ACKNOWLEDGMENTS

I'd like to thank the following people for their help and expertise in writing this book: Andy Jackson of the Exercise Company, for all his help and expertise, particularly concerning children's fitness; nutritionist Rozalind Gruben; osteopaths Paul Stamp and Helen Froggatt; Marilyn Creegor, for doing my make-up for the cover of this book; Penny Clarke, my editor; and Kate Ker, who taught me autogenic training and showed me how to relax while writing this book!

# NO SWEAT FITNESS FOR LIFE

Congratulations! You now have all the ingredients for being naturally fit and healthy for the rest of your life. I hope you are enjoying your new active daily routine and that you no longer think of exercise as hard work! This book will act as your 'personal trainer' for the years ahead. If you are ever in doubt about your programme, refer to the FITNESS TOOL-BOX, Parts one to five. Re-do the fitness tests on pages 45–7 and you should find a big improvement since you started the programme. Also re-do the questionnaires and you should have improved your score. I hope you are feeling more relaxed, healthier and full of energy.

Once your are confident that you are performing all the exercises in this book correctly, do not be afraid to incorporate them into other situations during the day. It doesn't matter where or when you choose to do an exercise, as long as you do it safely and with good technique. You should start to notice your body changing shape after just a few weeks. Remember – the more you do, the quicker you will get results. So do not waste any more time reading, get out there and get moving!

# CONTENTS

# INTRODUCTION

Wouldn't it be wonderful to be 'naturally fit'? To bound out of bed bursting with energy, to run for the bus without going red in the face, to look slim and sleek without having to diet and to boast a beautiful complexion without spending a fortune on cosmetics?

We all know about the bumper benefits of being fit. It can make you look better, feel better, cope better, live longer and can even, say the experts, do wonders for your sex life. Unfortunately, like dieting, exercising is one of the more tedious parts of life. It is hard for anyone to relish the thought of spending hard-earned money to go to sweaty gyms or cram-packed aerobics classes. Let's face it, most exercise regimes are boring. We all know we *should* do it, but wouldn't it be nicer if someone else could do the work for us!

*No Sweat Fitness* takes the sweat and effort out of getting fit. It is a unique programme that acts as your 'personal exercise trainer', showing you the easiest and simplest ways to get fit.

The reason that fitness has become such a major concern is that modern life is so sedentary. We have lost our ability to be 'naturally fit'. Genetically, our bodies are designed to be physically active. In terms of world history, it really isn't that long ago since we were out hunting and foraging for our food. At one time it was only the fittest and strongest who survived. Thankfully, we don't have to catch our own food any more and most of the physical challenges of life have been dissipated, but we still need to be 'fit' in order to survive the mental stresses of modern life. Without exercise, we become irritable and lethargic. It is a vicious circle: the less you do, the more unfit you become – which makes you feel tired and lethargic and so less inclined to do anything about it. 'I'm too tired' is one of the worst excuses for not exercising. The only way to break the circle is to get up and be active!

High technology is much to blame. Although it was originally designed to make our lives more 'efficient', it is actually damaging our health by making us inactive and fat. According to an obesity expert in the United States, people who switch from using a typewriter to a personal computer could gain up to half a stone in a year as they no longer even have to get up to consult a filing cabinet. Other fattening gadgets include remote-control televisions, elevators, dishwashers and extension phones, and even children, who used to be so active and full of energy, are playing less sport at school, spending more time slumped in front of the television or a computer game instead.

School PE was so unpleasant for many people that only three per cent of people in their 20s carry on with the sporting activities they did in their schooldays, and only one per cent continue them into their 30s. We have become a nation of couch potatoes and are growing physically old before our time. Indeed, another problem is the current trend for working at home. Although this saves you the stresses of commuting and office life, it also encourages you to be 'inactive' as there is no incentive for you to leave the house at all.

Ironically, instead of urging us to put more physical energy back into everyday life, the fitness industry is using high technology to trick us into thinking that exercise is not boring. Gymnasiums now look like large amusement arcades packed with gimmicky apparatus. You can row down a 'river' and be chased by sharks on a video screen in front of you, use a Stairmaster to climb up more stairs than there are in the Empire State Building, or be 'coached' by a talking weight machine called Wally. The fitness world is looking more like toy town every day, but unfortunately the novelty quickly wears off, and exercising soon becomes as tedious as ever.

However, get-fit resolutions are as fickle as promises to lose weight and there are so many excuses for breaking them – 'It's too cold… I'm too fat to go to a class… I've too much work to do… I'll start tomorrow.' It's amazing how some of the most determined people become spineless wimps when it comes to following a fitness programme. You see, exercise regimes do not work because, like diets, they are too rigid. You may start off very enthusiastically, but the chances are you will soon get bored – over three-quarters of people who join a health club do not renew their membership.

Short intense spells of exercise are like crash diets. They may have an effect in the short term, but in the long term all the benefits are lost and fat and flab will quickly return. For exercise to be of benefit it has to be long term. It has to be for life.

*No Sweat Fitness* works because it shows you how to incorporate exercise into your everyday routine. Boring tasks such as going to the supermarket, commuting to work or cleaning the kitchen can all be opportunities to tone up. A couple of minutes' movement here and there throughout the day can be just as beneficial as a full blown work-out.

*No Sweat Fitness* is the ideal modern and 'natural' approach. You can start getting fit the minute you read this book. There is no need for special equipment, clothing or hefty membership fees. It really is very simple – it is a new way to approach everyday tasks.

One of the main excuses for not sticking to a fitness programme is lack of time. Often there really do not seem to be enough hours in the day. If you have a high-powered job and are working around the clock you certainly will not want to spend valuable leisure time in a hot, sweaty gym. Alternatively, perhaps you are tied to the house looking after young children? Or maybe your job involves a lot of travelling so you find it hard to follow a fixed fitness routine? Whatever your lifestyle, *No Sweat Fitness* will be your personal trainer and show you how to get fit in a way that really suits you. It is an effortless and enjoyable approach to fitness that can be used by everyone of all ages, shapes and physical abilities.

Life itself is your natural gymnasium and everyday activities are all you need to get in shape. It is amazing how much time we waste. While standing at the bus-stop or waiting for the kettle to boil you could be toning up your arms or stretching out your legs. Instead of putting your clothes straight into the tumble drier, why not wring them by hand first, toning up the muscles in the chest and arms? When you are having a bath, why not use the warmth of the water to help you stretch out tight hamstrings? None of the movements are difficult to do, it is just a matter of learning how to incorporate them into your daily routine. They are not designed to pump you up into an Arnold Schwarzenegger, but will tone and streamline your body so that you will look sleeker and healthier than ever before.

*No Sweat Fitness* is brimming with ideas on how to increase your activity level. It is up to you how much or how little you do. But once you start to shape up you will have a whole new boost of energy and may suddenly be inspired to take up something new, whether this be riding along the beach at dawn or doing t'ai chi at sunset on your lawn.

As a counterbalance to all this new activity, this book also includes a section called NO SWEAT RELAXATION which shows you how to unwind. If weight loss is a concern, you should find that you lose a lot of unwanted fat just by increasing your activity level, but I have also included a section called NO SWEAT NUTRITION, an easy-to-follow plan of healthy eating habits which will keep you slim for life.

So whatever your reasons for wanting to get fit, I hope *No Sweat Fitness* brings back natural movement into your life. I know you will feel better for it.

# THE NO SWEAT FITNESS PLAN

Congratulations! You are now on the way to being naturally fit and slim – for the rest of your life. The *No Sweat Fitness* plan began the minute you started reading this book. There is no need to go to sweaty gyms or cram-packed aerobics classes and you can save money by not having to pay membership fees or for fancy work-out clothing. Life itself is a free gymnasium and everyday activities will keep you trim. It doesn't matter what your age, shape or physical ability, the *No Sweat Fitness* plan is so simple that anyone can do it. So let's get started.

## TAILOR-MADE FITNESS

*No Sweat Fitness* is a unique fitness programme which can be tailor-made to suit your individual needs. This book is your personal exercise trainer and with the help of questionnaires and simple do-it-yourself fitness tests it will show you exactly what you personally need to do to get into shape.

Although you will find useful tips and information throughout the book, it has been divided into easy-to-follow sections so that you can dip straight in and find the one most appropriate for you.

## A FIRM FOUNDATION: PARTS 1–5

The foundations of *No Sweat Fitness* are clearly laid down in sections 1–5 and apply to everybody – please don't skip them as they are vital for your long-term success! In Part 1 you will discover just how active (or inactive, as the case may be) you really are, and in Part 2 you will learn all about fitness and what you can achieve on the *No Sweat Fitness* programme. Part 3 shows you how to warm up and cool down safely, while in Part 4 you will learn the principles of good technique so that you will get the best results and Part 5 gets you walking yourself thin. Although they won't take very long to read, they are full of useful tips and advice. Look at them as a 'fitness tool-box', full of 'tools' enabling you to sculpt your body into perfect shape. Once equipped with these, it is up to you what effect you want to create. You will quickly be able to turn to the most appropriate chapters. And remember, this 'tool-box' is always there as a back-up if you ever need help in progressing or changing your programme.

# THE NO SWEAT FITNESS QUESTIONNAIRE

Answer the following questions as honestly as possible. Remember, this is not a competition and there is no 'right' or 'wrong' answer. Then turn to ANSWERS opposite to discover which sections in this book are most appropriate for you.

1. Would you describe your job as stressful?

   A Yes, very
   B Moderately so
   C No

2. How do you travel to work?

   A Bus, car, tube or train
   B Foot
   C Bicycle
   D Don't travel to work (i.e. based at home)

3. At the end of the day how would you describe yourself?

   A Exhausted
   B Tired
   C Tense and wound-up
   D Feeling fairly good

4. Do you have children?

   A Yes
   B No

5. How would you describe yourself?

   A A sociable person who likes to do things in groups
   B A loner

6. Would you describe yourself as competitive?

   A Yes
   B No

7. Tick any of the following reasons why you want to get fit:

   A To lose weight
   B For more energy
   C To keep up with your kids
   D To combat stress

8. How much time are your prepared to dedicate to getting 'fit'?

   A Nothing on a regular basis
   B Less than ten minutes, three times per week
   C 10–20 minutes, three times per week
   D 20–40 minutes, three times per week
   E 40–60 minutes, three times per week
   F More than an hour, three or more times per week

# ANSWERS

1. A and B Turn to THE WALKING PROGRAMME, THE WORKER'S WORK-OUT and NO SWEAT RELAXATION.

If your job is highly stressful you will find the stretching and mobility movements in THE WORKER'S WORK-OUT very useful for alleviating physical tension. You should also increase the amount of walking or aerobic exercise that you do as this is excellent for relieving stress (see THE WALKING PROGRAMME). Also see NO SWEAT RELAXATION.

2. A Turn to THE WALKING PROGRAMME and THE
WORKER'S WORK-OUT.
B Turn to THE WALKING PROGRAMME, NO SWEAT
SPORT and THE WORKER'S WORK-OUT.
C Turn to NO SWEAT SPORT and the WORKER'S WORK-
OUT.
D Turn to THE HOME WORK-OUT and THE WALKING
PROGRAMME. If you are looking after kids, turn to THE FAMILY
WORK-OUT.

Travelling to work is an ideal opportunity to tone up. For movements you
can do sitting on the train, bus or in the car see THE WORKER'S
WORK-OUT. Also see THE WALKING PROGRAMME. If you
already cycle or walk to work you may enjoy trying some of the other sports
in NO SWEAT SPORT.

3. A Turn to NO SWEAT NUTRITION, NO SWEAT RE-
LAXATION and THE WALKING PROGRAMME.
B Turn to NO SWEAT NUTRITION, NO SWEAT RE-
LAXATION, THE HOME WORK-OUT and THE WALKING
PROGRAMME.
C Turn to NO SWEAT SPORT, THE WALKING PRO-
GRAMME and NO SWEAT RELAXATION.
D Turn to THE HOME WORK-OUT, NO SWEAT SPORT and
THE WALKING PROGRAMME.

A lack of energy is a common complaint in our stressful society. Many
people say that they are too 'tired' to exercise. If you are tired through stress,
however, rather than through lack of sleep, a hangover or an illness, one of
the best pep-ups is to go for a long walk or do something physical. Your
diet can also affect your energy levels.

4. A Turn to THE FAMILY WORK-OUT.

Although looking after children can be exhausting, it is actually an excellent
way to keep fit. THE FAMILY WORK-OUT section is full of movements
designed to keep you and your children in trim.

5. A Turn to NO SWEAT SPORT or THE FAMILY WORK-OUT
(if you have kids).

If you do not like doing things on your own, you may prefer the social
element of taking up one of the sports listed in the NO SWEAT SPORT

section. Alternatively, if you have children why not join in with their fun fitness games or take them on an active outing at the weekend?

6. A   Turn to THE NO SWEAT FITNESS TESTS and NO SWEAT SPORT.
   B   Turn to THE NO SWEAT FITNESS TESTS.

If you are competitive by nature, you will enjoy doing the fitness tests on pp45–7. You may also like to try some of the competitive sports in the NO SWEAT SPORT section. If you are not competitive you should still do the fitness tests as they are an important way of seeing how your fitness improves.

7. A   Turn to NO SWEAT NUTRITION and THE WALKING PROGRAMME.
   B   Turn to NO SWEAT NUTRITION, NO SWEAT RE-LAXATION and THE WALKING PROGRAMME.
   C   Turn to THE FAMILY WORK-OUT.
   D   Turn to NO SWEAT RELAXATION and THE WALKING PROGRAMME.

If you want to lose weight you need to do aerobic exercise, and THE WALKING PROGRAMME is an ideal way to start. You also need to look at some of the diet recommendations in NO SWEAT NUTRITION.

A lack of energy can be caused by many things. Check that your diet is good in the NO SWEAT NUTRITION section. You may also lack energy if you are under stress so read the NO SWEAT RELAXATION section. There is a lot of truth in the old adage that 'energy creates energy'. THE WALKING PROGRAMME is an excellent way to perk yourself up.

Looking after kids can be very tiring! Do THE FAMILY WORK-OUT and make sure that you all stay fit and have fun together.

Stress is a major problem in our society and something that you really need to start dealing with *now*. The NO SWEAT RELAXATION chapter is full of tips on how to stay calm and collected. Aerobic exercise is also an excellent way to alleviate stress so make sure you follow THE WALKING PROGRAMME.

8. A   Turn to THE WALKING PROGRAMME.
   B, C and D   Turn to THE WALKING PROGRAMME and either THE HOME WORK-OUT (if you are based at home) or THE WORKER'S WORK-OUT.

E and F   Turn to THE WALKING PROGRAMME, THE HOME WORK-OUT (if you are based at home), THE WORKER'S WORK-OUT and NO SWEAT SPORT.

*No Sweat Fitness* will not take up a lot of your time. To build up a good base for fitness, you should start with THE WALKING PROGRAMME. This can easily be incorporated into everyday life so you do not need to feel that you are 'dedicating' any particular time at all.

Once you have built up a solid fitness base with THE WALKING PROGRAMME you can start doing the movements in other sections of the book such as THE HOME WORK-OUT and THE WORKER'S WORK-OUT. These use snatched moments throughout the day so again you won't feel like you are dedicating a lot of time to getting fit.

When your body starts to shape up you will have more energy and will feel more inclined to become involved in extra activities. At this stage you may like to look at the NO SWEAT SPORT chapter.


## LONG-LASTING RESULTS

*No Sweat Fitness* can work very quickly. After only the first week or two you should feel more energetic, self-confident and streamlined. The more you do, the more your muscles will tone, your stomach will flatten and your general appearance and figure improve. The movements are not designed to pump you up into a Mr Universe but they will give you a naturally athletic-looking body. However, if it has taken years of inactivity to turn you into a lifeless blob, you can't expect to reverse the process overnight! There is no need to hurry. Every day will see some improvement. This is not a crash fitness programme – this is fitness for life. The only successful fitness plan is the one you adopt for ever. Take your time and enjoy your new active way of life. Once you start doing these movements you will see how easy they are and be surprised that you never thought of doing them before. Our bodies are designed to be active and you will feel so much more alert once you get your system going again.

Now is the time to start!

# THE FITNESS TOOL-BOX

# PART ONE

## ENERGY!

*REMEMBER! This section is part of your FITNESS TOOL-BOX. Don't skip it! You need to read this section in order to be fully equipped to do the NO SWEAT FITNESS PROGRAMME.*

## BODY IMAGE

In the first part of the *No Sweat Fitness* plan you don't physically have to do anything at all! All you need to do is start thinking thin and boosting your self-image.

What do you think of your body shape? Do you feel like a fat ugly blimp or are you quite happy with your figure? The way you visualise yourself is often reflected in your appearance but it is actually very hard to be honest with yourself about how you really look and if you are the sort of person who refuses to have your photo taken, you may be suffering from a poor body image. This is very dangerous and often closely linked with eating disorders. When a group of anorexics at the Royal Free Hospital in London, for example, were asked to look in the mirror and visually estimate their shape, many of them overestimated by as much as 50 per cent. Someone with a healthy body image should not be more than half an inch out.

Unfortunately, the fitness industry is cashing in on this vulnerability. Even if you are the 'ideal' weight medically, you will always find a fitness instructor ready to insist that you have at least another stone to lose. Most people who go to a gymnasium come out feeling fat and flabby after their initial consultation. Surrounded by a roomful of body beautifuls, most of us feel self-conscious and physically inadequate.

It is easy to become obsessed with the 'perfect' body. Our image of this ideal is partly developed by the media but is also dependent on social and economic factors. In Africa, for example, 'thin' is ugly as it is associated with poverty and starvation. Daughters from wealthy families are actually sent to 'fattening houses' instead of finishing schools, as the plumper the wife, the bigger the status symbol! And it is an ideal which has been around for thousands of years. We in the West are much more fickle, though, and keep changing our minds. In the 1950s, for example, a full, curvaceous figure was desirable for women whereas only a decade later, the thin, emaciated 'Twiggy' look was the ultimate. Today, however, the 'fit and healthy' look is what people of both sexes are aiming at, so the pendulum is beginning to swing back again.

## REALISTIC EXPECTATIONS

By following the natural everyday movements in this book, you will greatly improve your body shape and will look and feel better than you have ever done before. However, you must be realistic about how much you can hope to change your particular body shape. Genetically, there are actually three main body types – mesomorphs (muscular), ectomorphs (light) and endomorphs (rounded) – but, as most people have characteristics from more than one type, this sort of classification is not very helpful. The important point to remember always is that it is impossible to change your skeletal frame. No amount of exercise or dieting can ever change short stubby legs into long lean ones! Similarly, a man who is naturally slender, with narrow shoulders and hips and long skinny limbs, will find it very hard – if not impossible – to build himself up into Mr Universe proportions, although he will be able to strengthen and build up his physique so that he looks strong and athletic. This book will help everyone streamline their shape and improve their posture so that even if they haven't actually grown they will tend to 'look' taller and slimmer.

# THINK THIN!

Whatever your body type, it is important that you improve your self-image. If you have a poor body image you will feel unattractive and lack self-esteem, being embarrassed to move and not using your body properly or efficiently. The unconscious, creative part of your brain is easily convinced that something is true if you repeatedly keep telling it so. If you keep thinking yourself 'fat', your brain will eventually believe you and so you will start behaving accordingly, moving slowly and lethargically to conserve energy. Similarly, if you think of yourself as 'puny' and 'feeble' you may well start acting like a wimp!

Take a look at the way thin people behave and you'll notice that they seem to do everything with much more energy and vigour than heavier individuals. Even if you are on the plump side, start thinking thin and make a conscious effort to move around as though you were a stone or two lighter. Increasing your energy output is a vital ingredient in the *No Sweat Fitness* plan. Once you start approaching everything with more gusto, you will quickly begin to change shape. Likewise, if you have always thought of yourself as feeble or frail, start imagining yourself as someone who is powerful and athletic. Stride out with confidence! The essence of 'strength' really does come from within and with the movements in this book improving your posture and muscle tone, there is no reason to think of yourself as 'feeble' ever again!

# HOW ACTIVE ARE YOU?

Answer the following questions to find out how active your lifestyle really is. Remember to answer honestly – this is not a competition! Then turn to pp29–32 to find out how you have scored and what your current activity rating is.

1. Where do you live?

    A  In a house (i.e. with one or more flights of stairs)
    B  In a ground-floor flat or bungalow

    C In a first-floor (or above) flat – you use the stairs
    D In a first-floor (or above) flat – you use the lift

2. What is your main form of transport?

    A A car or motorbike
    B A bicycle
    C Walking
    D Public transport (e.g. bus, train or tube)

3. How much of your journey to work is spent on foot or on a bicycle?

    A Not applicable (i.e. I stay at home)
    B Less than five minutes
    C 5–10 minutes
    D 10–20 minutes
    E 20–30 minutes
    F More than 30 minutes

4. When was the last time you exercised or played sport on a regular basis?

    A More than five years ago
    B More than a year ago
    C A few months ago
    D Currently exercise or play sport regularly

5. Score three points for every time you do any sport or exercise in a week. Include walking here if it lasts longer than 15 minutes.

6. What sort of holiday do you usually take?

    A Don't go on holiday
    B Beach holiday
    C Combination of beach and activities (e.g. waterskiing, wind-surfing etc.)
    D Sightseeing holiday
    E Activity holiday (e.g. cycling, sailing, horseriding, skiing, wind-surfing, tennis etc.)
    F Walking or hiking holiday
    G Adventure holiday (e.g. safari, white-water rafting, canoeing etc.)

7. At lunchtime what do you usually do?

    A Stay where you are (i.e. eat lunch at your desk)
    B Go out to buy sandwiches
    C Go out for a business lunch
    D Go shopping
    E Go for a walk
    F Play sport or exercise

8. Approximately how many hours during the working day do you spend sitting down?

    A More than eight
    B 5–8 hours
    C 2–4 hours
    D Less than two hours

9. How would you describe yourself?

    A Hyperactive or always rushing around
    B Moderately energetic
    C Slow and calm
    D Tired and lethargic

10. Score two points for each of the following that you do regularly at the weekend.

    A Gardening
    B Take the children out
    C Play sport or exercise
    D Go for long walks
    E Housework
    F Other physical activity (e.g. DIY, lifting boxes etc.)

11. If you have to run 100 m for a bus or a train, how would you describe yourself?

    A Not able to run 100 m for a bus or a train
    B Red in the face, panting and exhausted
    C Hot and sweaty and breathing heavily
    D Slightly warmer than usual and breathing a little heavier
    E Not affected

12. If you go to work, how do you tackle going from floor to floor?

    A Run up or down the stairs
    B Walk up or down the stairs
    C Take the lift
    D Office is on ground-level

13. If you had to run up two flights of stairs, how would you feel?

    A Unable to
    B Would have to stop halfway
    C Exhausted, red in the face and very breathless
    D A little warm and pink in the face
    E Fine

14. How do you do your weekly shopping?

    A Charge round with a basket and walk home
    B Charge round with a basket and drive/bus home
    C Push a trolley round and walk home
    D Push a trolley round and drive/bus home
    E Send someone to do your shopping for you

15. Faced with a long escalator what do you do?

    A Stand on it
    B Walk up it
    C Run up it

16. When was the last time you went for a 30-minute or longer walk?

    A Cannot remember
    B Years ago
    C Months ago
    D A few weeks ago
    E Last week
    F Yesterday

17. It is six o'clock in the evening, you have just got home and realise you are out of milk. The nearest shop is half a mile away. What do you do?

    A Forget about the milk
    B Drive to the shop
    C Send your child or partner to buy the milk

D  Catch the bus
E  Walk to the shop
F  Run or cycle to the shop

18. Do you have a dog?

A  No
B  Yes, and I walk it regularly
C  Yes, and I walk it occasionally or at weekends
D  Yes, but someone else takes it for walks

19. Your favourite song is played on the radio. What do you do?

A  Turn up the sound and start dancing around the room
B  Turn up the sound and start tapping your feet or slowly moving around
C  Don't move but sing along
D  You don't listen to the radio

## ANSWERS

1. a = 2  b = 0  c = 1  d = 0
2. a = 0  b = 2  c = 3  d = 0
3. a = 0  b = 0  c = 1  d = 2  e = 3  f = 4
4. a = 0  b = 0  c = 1  d = 2
5. Score 3 points for every time you do any sport or exercise in a week. Include walking if it lasts longer than 20 minutes
6. a = 0  b = 1  c = 2  d = 1  e = 3  f = 3  g = 3
7. a = 0  b = 1  c = 0  d = 1  e = 3  f = 4
8. a = 0  b = 1  c = 2  d = 3
9. a = 3  b = 2  c = 1  d = 0
10. Score 2 points for each tick
11. a = 0  b = 1  c = 2  d = 3  e = 4
12. a = 4  b = 2  c = 0  d = 0
13. a = 0  b = 1  c = 2  d = 3  e = 4
14. a = 4  b = 3  c = 3  d = 1  e = 0
15. a = 0  b = 3  c = 4
16. a = 0  b = 0  c = 1  d = 2  e = 3  f = 4
17. a = 0  b = 1  c = 0  d = 1  e = 3  f = 4
18. a = 0  b = 2  c = 1  d = 0
19. a = 4  b = 2  c = 0  d = 0

# ACTIVITY RATING

Add up the total number of points you scored to see how active you really are. Don't worry if you have a low rating now. If you try this questionnaire again in a few weeks time you should see that your activity score has improved quite dramatically!

## OVER 40 POINTS

Congratulations! You are a very active, energetic person and will no doubt enjoy all the new everyday movements you will learn in this book. As well as THE HOME WORK-OUT and THE WORKER'S WORK-OUT, you may also be interested in learning a new sport (see NO SWEAT SPORT) or checking to see that your diet is good (see NO SWEAT NUTRITION). If you have children, you should also look at THE FAMILY WORK-OUT and encourage your kids to be as active as you!

> *REMEMBER! Make sure you read Sections 1–5 thoroughly before you start on any of the other sections. This is your FITNESS TOOL-BOX which will enable you to get the best results from the programme as a whole.*

## 22–39 POINTS

You have great potential for being superactive! Your score shows that you are already active and energetic in many ways and this book will show you how to boost your activity level a little higher in order to become fitter and healthier. You are probably missing many occasions when you could be burning up calories and using your body strength. Think of simple ways to be more energetic such as striding out when you walk, running up the stairs and carrying the shopping home! You may have missed out on points because you have always thought you haven't got time to be active. The *No Sweat Fitness* programme is ideal for you as it will show you how to tailor-make a fitness plan to suit your lifestyle. For example, if you seem to spend most of your day behind a desk, turn to THE WORKER'S WORK-OUT. If you stay at home with the kids or work from home, turn to THE HOME WORK-OUT. Whatever your lifestyle, you will find plenty of help in getting fit.

> *REMEMBER! Make sure you read Sections 1–5 thoroughly before you start on any of the other sections. This is your FITNESS TOOL-BOX which will enable you to get the best results from the programme as a whole.*

## 10–21 POINTS

You have your 'active' moments, but you are missing a lot of natural opportunity to keep fit. Don't worry if you haven't scored a lot of points the first time you do this questionnaire. You have plenty of time to increase your activity level and *No Sweat Fitness* will show you exactly how. For example, if you usually drive to work, park the car further away than usual and walk the last few hundred metres. Or if you are based at home, get up and move about as much as possible – turn up the radio when you hear your favourite record and dance about! You will also find THE WALKING PROGRAMME an excellent way to boost your energy.

> *REMEMBER! Make sure you read Sections 1–5 thoroughly before you start on any of the other sections. This is your FITNESS TOOL-BOX which will enable you to get the best results from the programme as a whole.*

## 0–9 POINTS

I'm sure you realise that you could be a lot more active! But even if your score does come under this category, don't despair. Some of the biggest couch potatoes become the fittest and most active people when they realise how easy the *No Sweat Fitness* programme is. Remember, this is fitness without the pain and agony of a rigorous routine. You don't have to strip off into a leotard and jump up and down in an aerobics class! All you have to do is follow the guidelines in this book and find simple ways to make your life more active. And the more you do, the less effort it will become. Yes, you may have to stop halfway when you first walk up the stairs, but in a few weeks' time you will be doing it with ease. Remember – ENERGY

CREATES ENERGY, so get moving! Make sure you follow the energy plan below. Look at the points you've scored in the questions above and see how these could be improved. Think about simple things such as walking up the stairs instead of waiting for the lift, walking to a sandwich shop further away than usual at lunchtime and getting up to change TV channels by hand rather than using the remote control. All this will have a snowball effect as the more you do, the better you will feel, and so will feel encouraged to keep moving. Try this questionnaire again in a few weeks' time and I'm sure you will be surprised to see how much your score has shot up.

> *REMEMBER! Make sure you read Sections 1–5 thoroughly before you start on any of the other sections. This is your FITNESS TOOL-BOX which will enable you to get the best results from the programme as a whole.*

# ENERGY!

Now is the time to get your system fired up. Spend the next week doing everything in a higher gear than usual. For example, if you usually take the lift, walk up the stairs instead. If you are already used to walking up the stairs, now start running up them. *No Sweat Fitness* is all about progression. It doesn't matter how slowly you take things. The only person you are competing against is yourself.

Think of ways that you personally can improve your energy output. Walk everywhere faster than usual, and start becoming aware of every little movement you make, be it standing up from a chair or picking up a cup of coffee. When you walk, feel that you are pushing the ground away from underneath your feet. Think of your body as a powerful machine and yourself as an athlete. Be proud of the way your body moves. Visualise the muscles contracting and relaxing whenever you do something, be it opening a door or a can of cat food or stepping into the bath. Put more physical effort into everything – jump up and change the TV channel instead of using the remote control, rush round the supermarket with a basket instead of sauntering round with a trolley, and be the first on the dance floor at a party!

Energy creates energy, and by moving around positively your circulation will improve, you will burn up more calories and will soon start to feel revitalised.

## ENERGY EVALUATION

One of the best ways to motivate yourself is to keep a record of how energetic you are each day. In the tables below are a list of activities that enable you to use up physical energy. Don't worry if these don't all apply to you. There is space at the bottom of this list to add other activities that personally apply. Perhaps you use up a lot of physical energy looking after an elderly or handicapped person? Or maybe you have a dog which needs walking (or have a particularly active sex life!)? But whichever activities you choose to include in your list, award yourself points each day as to how 'energetically' you think you approached them.

   5 = maximum energy
   4 = very energetic
   3 = energetic
   2 = lightly energetic
   1 = lethargic
   0 = no energy

For example, if you think you were 'very energetic' when you commuted to work, award yourself 4 points. Or if you think you were physically 'lethargic' all day at work, award yourself none. Remember, the only person you are competing against is yourself. It doesn't matter if you score 0 in Week 1, as long as you score at least 1 in Week 2!

## ENERGY EXPENDITURE: WEEK 1

|  | Mon | Tue | Wed | Thur | Fri | Sat | Sun |
|---|---|---|---|---|---|---|---|
| HOUSEWORK |  |  |  |  |  |  |  |
| TRAVELLING TO WORK |  |  |  |  |  |  |  |
| SHOPPING |  |  |  |  |  |  |  |
| GARDENING/WASHING CAR |  |  |  |  |  |  |  |
| SPORT |  |  |  |  |  |  |  |
| PLAYING WITH KIDS |  |  |  |  |  |  |  |
| SOCIALISING! |  |  |  |  |  |  |  |
| WORKING |  |  |  |  |  |  |  |
| Filing |  |  |  |  |  |  |  |
| Lifting boxes |  |  |  |  |  |  |  |
| Rushing around on your feet |  |  |  |  |  |  |  |
| (Add other activities that apply to you) |  |  |  |  |  |  |  |
| DAILY TOTAL |  |  |  |  |  |  |  |

WEEK 1 TOTAL =

## ENERGY EXPENDITURE: WEEK 2

Week 1 was your base energy level. Try to improve on the score this week.

|  | Mon | Tue | Wed | Thur | Fri | Sat | Sun |
|---|---|---|---|---|---|---|---|
| HOUSEWORK |  |  |  |  |  |  |  |
| TRAVELLING TO WORK |  |  |  |  |  |  |  |
| SHOPPING |  |  |  |  |  |  |  |
| GARDENING/WASHING CAR |  |  |  |  |  |  |  |
| SPORT |  |  |  |  |  |  |  |
| PLAYING WITH KIDS |  |  |  |  |  |  |  |
| SOCIALISING! |  |  |  |  |  |  |  |
| WORKING |  |  |  |  |  |  |  |
| Filing |  |  |  |  |  |  |  |
| Lifting boxes |  |  |  |  |  |  |  |
| Rushing around on your feet |  |  |  |  |  |  |  |
| (Add other activities that apply to you) |  |  |  |  |  |  |  |
| DAILY TOTAL |  |  |  |  |  |  |  |

WEEK 2 TOTAL =

## ENERGY EXPENDITURE: WEEK 3

Try to improve on the score from Week 2.

| | Mon | Tue | Wed | Thur | Fri | Sat | Sun |
|---|---|---|---|---|---|---|---|
| HOUSEWORK | | | | | | | |
| TRAVELLING TO WORK | | | | | | | |
| SHOPPING | | | | | | | |
| GARDENING/WASHING CAR | | | | | | | |
| SPORT | | | | | | | |
| PLAYING WITH KIDS | | | | | | | |
| SOCIALISING! | | | | | | | |
| WORKING Filing Lifting boxes Rushing around on your feet (Add other activities that apply to you) | | | | | | | |
| DAILY TOTAL | | | | | | | |

WEEK 3 TOTAL =

## ENERGY EXPENDITURE: WEEK 4

Your energy expenditure should now be improving. Really 'go for it' in everything you do this week and you should see your score shoot up.

| | Mon | Tue | Wed | Thur | Fri | Sat | Sun |
|---|---|---|---|---|---|---|---|
| HOUSEWORK | | | | | | | |
| TRAVELLING TO WORK | | | | | | | |
| SHOPPING | | | | | | | |
| GARDENING/WASHING CAR | | | | | | | |
| SPORT | | | | | | | |
| PLAYING WITH KIDS | | | | | | | |
| SOCIALISING! | | | | | | | |
| WORKING Filing Lifting boxes Rushing around on your feet (Add other activities that apply to you) | | | | | | | |
| DAILY TOTAL | | | | | | | |

WEEK 4 TOTAL =

Well done! By following this subjective energy evaluation you should have discovered ways to improve your activity level. You may find it useful to continue using this chart for at least another week, as it will get you into the habit of thinking ACTIVE. I also use it at special times of the year such as Christmas, when it is so easy to be a couch potato.

# PART TWO

## NO SWEAT FITNESS

*REMEMBER! Part Two is part of your FITNESS TOOL-BOX. Don't skip it! You need to read this section carefully in order to be fully equipped to do the NO SWEAT FITNESS programme.*

## DEFINITION OF FITNESS

If you have bought this book and read this far you have obviously decided you want or need to get fit. But what does the word 'fitness' actually mean? Everyone has their own interpretation. A marathon runner, for example, has very different 'fitness' objectives to someone who just wants to be able to catch the number 79 bus!

When we talk about 'fitness' we have to ask 'Fit for what?' In *No Sweat Fitness* we are concerned with health-related fitness. This book will not prepare you to run a marathon (although it may give you the confidence to train for one) but it will enable you to catch the bus and still feel full of energy when you get to work. It will also give you more energy and confidence to cope with the mental and physical demands of everyday life, allowing you to enjoy other 'active' pursuits, be it windsurfing on holiday or playing 'tag' with the kids at weekends. When you are 'fit', life suddenly becomes so much easier. You will no longer be huffing and puffing at the slightest exertion and won't fall asleep on the sofa before the nine o'clock news.

Physical fitness is only part of *No Sweat Fitness*. You can be physically 'fit' but still unhealthy. Many athletes, for example, do so much training that they overstress their bodies and are no longer 'healthy'. But *No Sweat Fitness* will get you fit *and* healthy. Reading this book is just the beginning. *No Sweat Fitness* encourages you to be active for the rest of your life. So don't hurry! If you can not walk a whole mile now, never mind. In six weeks, 12 weeks or however many it takes, you will. We will all get there in time! There is no need to compete. Take things at your own pace.

To be 'fit' in the healthiest sense you also need a good diet and to be able to cope with stress, aspects we will be looking at later, but in this part we are going to look at the 'physical' aspects of fitness, and for the purposes of this book, 'physical fitness' can be divided into three major components – aerobic fitness, muscular strength/endurance, and flexibility.


# AEROBIC FITNESS

BENEFITS:   REDUCES BODY FAT
            REDUCES BLOOD FATS (CHOLESTEROL AND GLYCERIDES)
            REDUCES THE RISK OF CORONARY HEART DISEASE
            REDUCES STRESS
            ELEVATES MOOD ('RUNNER'S HIGH')
            LOWERS BLOOD PRESSURE OF HYPERTENSIVES
            HELPS CONTROL DIABETES/GLUCOSE INTOLERANCE
            INCREASES ENERGY FOR EVERYDAY TASKS
            HELPS YOU GIVE UP SMOKING

From a health point of view, aerobic fitness (also known as cardiorespiratory fitness) is the most important part of your fitness programme. Not many people die from weak quadriceps (thigh muscles) or tight hamstrings (back of leg muscles) but cardiovascular disease is the biggest killer in the western world. Aerobic exercise strengthens the heart and can help prevent coronary heart disease.

'Aerobic' literally means 'with oxygen', and when you exercise aerobically you have to breathe in enough oxygen to supply your muscles so that they can continue working for a length of time. It is rhythmic exercise which uses the large muscle groups, at low tension, for an extended period of time, and aerobic activities include jogging, running, walking, swimming, cycling, rowing, cross-country skiing, dancing and exercise classes to music. All of these will strengthen your heart so that it is able to pump more blood round the body with each beat. Your heart is, after all, a muscle and aerobic exercise will make it grow bigger and stronger so that it does not have to work so hard, therefore reducing the number of times it has to beat per minute. Indeed, your lung capacity will also increase, making them more efficient in transporting oxygen, so that by improving your aerobic fitness, you will have more energy for everyday tasks and simple activities such as walking up the stairs will seem so much easier.

There are many ways of incorporating aerobic exercise into everyday life, such as cycling to work, dancing, walking or taking the children swimming at weekends. In order to strengthen your heart and lungs, you should aim to do some sort of aerobic exercise two to three times a week, preferably on alternate days. Make sure you keep moving for 15 minutes, although if you are very unfit you may need to build up to this slowly. As aerobic exercise is the best way of burning off body fat – fat being the main source of fuel in this type of activity – you may want to use it as a way to lose weight. In this case, try to build up longer sessions (20–30 minutes) more frequently (four or five times a week), and also look at THE WALKING PROGRAMME for further details.

You will know when you are exercising aerobically as you will start breathing harder and getting warmer. If you are not used to this type of exercise you will probably find that a brisk walk is enough to put your heart rate up. This does not mean you need to turn scarlet and be soaked with sweat! In fact, you want to avoid exercising too vigorously or there will not be enough oxygen for your body to burn fat and you will very quickly fatigue and have to stop exercising altogether! Fast, intense exercise such as sprinting (known as 'anaer-obic' – that is, without oxygen) is only appropriate for well-con-ditioned athletes who need this stop-start type of activity as part of their training. However, if you have high blood or heart problems this anaerobic exercise could be dangerous and is not part of the *No Sweat Fitness* plan as it does not help you burn fat or have any additional health benefits.

## CHECKING THAT YOU ARE EXERCISING AEROBICALLY

You should know that you are exercising aerobically by simple signs such as a slight breathlessness, an increase in body temperature and a pinker skin tone. If you feel so breathless that you could not hold a conversation, you are exercising too vigorously. As you get fitter, you will, of course, be able to increase the intensity and duration of the activity, but make sure you never go beyond being *comfortably* out of breath.

# MUSCULAR STRENGTH AND ENDURANCE

BENEFITS: IMPROVES POSTURE
HELPS LOW BACK PAIN
REDUCES THE CHANCE OF OSTEOPOROSIS (BRITTLE BONES)
GIVES YOU MORE ENERGY
HELPS YOU CARRY OUT EVERYDAY TASKS

Muscular strength and endurance are actually two different components of fitness, although for the purpose of this book they can be grouped together. Muscular strength refers to the maximum force a muscle can exert to overcome a resistance. Muscular endurance, on the other hand, is the ability of a muscle to overcome resistance for an extended period of time. For strength training you need to use heavy weights and low repetitions. For muscular endurance training you use light weights and lots of repetitions.

Women often shy away from strength training as they are worried that they will end up with big bulky muscles. Rest assured. This book will not pump you up into an Arnold Schwarzenegger! The *No Sweat Fitness* movements are more endurance-based and designed to increase muscle tone and definition rather than to increase muscle size. They do not involve using heavy weights but teach you to rely on your own body weight, and use light everyday objects such as oranges or tins of baked beans!

One of the most important concepts of strength and endurance training is the need for 'progression'. The following fable illustrates this point.

Thousands of years ago there was a farmer who one day had to lift a baby calf out of harm's way. His wife was watching him and complimented him on his strength. The farmer was secretly proud of his strength so every night he would sneak down to see the calf and lift it triumphantly above his head. A few months later he had an argument with his brother who called him a coward and insulted his pride. His wife defended him by saying he could lift a whole calf above his head. The brother laughed and said that was no big deal, so could he. They went down to the barn to see this calf – which by now was a full-grown cow – and the brother tried to lift it but could not move it so much as an inch above the ground. The farmer then stepped forward and lifted the full-grown cow right above his head. The argument was clearly won.

The reason that the farmer could lift a full-grown cow was that he had trained for it over the months by gradually lifting heavier and heavier weights (i.e. the growing cow).

Don't worry, you are not going to have to lift any cows in *No Sweat Fitness*! You will, however, need to keep increasing the weight or the number of repetitions you do in order to improve the strength and endurance of your muscles. For this reason each movement in this book gives you a target to work to.

# FLEXIBILITY

BENEFITS: IMPROVES POSTURE
HELPS PREVENT INJURIES
HELPS PROMOTE CIRCULATION
HELPS PREVENT AND RELIEVE LOWER-BACK PAIN
REDUCES MUSCLE TENSION AND SO MAKES YOU FEEL BETTER
HELPS YOU CARRY OUT EVERYDAY TASKS

This book is full of stretching movements designed to improve your flexibility. The most important thing to remember is that you must warm up *before* you stretch. You need to 'hold' the stretch for a minimum of 6–10 seconds but you will be given precise instructions with each movement.

To improve your flexibility you need to stretch every day. As this is one of the most pleasurable and soothing types of exercise this should not be too daunting! Aim to ease gently into a stretch until you feel a little bit of tension. This tension is caused by what is known as the 'stretch reflex', the body's way of protecting itself. When you try to stretch a muscle, the brain makes the muscle contract in order to prevent it from being overextended or damaged. The more you try to force the stretch, the stronger the stretch reflex fires and the more tension and even pain you will feel in the muscle. This is why you should avoid any jerky, bouncing movements known as 'ballistic stretching'. Instead, you should ease gently into the stretch until you feel a mild sensation of tension. If you hold the stretch quietly in that position, the stretch reflex will back off as it thinks the muscle is out of danger. This takes about 6–10 seconds, allowing you to develop the stretch by gently easing into it further until you feel some mild tension again. If you take things gently and sneak up on the stretch reflex, you can stretch for up to 30 seconds or more with excellent results.

# SELF-ASSESSMENT

Before you start the *No Sweat Fitness* programme it is useful to do some basic fitness tests. Don't worry – this is not a competition and these tests are not trying to determine whether you are 'good' or 'bad'. Use them as a guideline to see how much you improve over the next few weeks.

The first thing you need to assess is whether it is safe for you to do this exercise programme. Make sure you read the following points carefully.

> *Before starting this or any exercise programme, you should consult your GP if:*
> *you are pregnant;*

*you suffer from diabetes, high blood pressure, epilepsy, high cholesterol, elevated blood lipids, or any cardiovascular problems;*
*you are over 35 and have not been regularly exercising in the last year;*
*you suffer from back problems or are still recovering from an injury;*
*you are prone to dizziness, headaches, or fainting;*
*you have a family history of coronary heart disease;*
*you are a heavy smoker;*
*you are taking drugs or medication at the moment or are still recuperating from an illness or operation.*

If none of the above applies you can do the simple fitness tests below. Try to do these when you have just come back from a walk so your body is warm. Be careful not to overstrain yourself.

## BODY FAT

### THE PINCH AN INCH TEST!

The only way to assess your body fat percentage accurately is to have it tested by a health professional with callipers or by hydrostatic weighing (total immersion in water). It is possible, however, to give yourself a rough assessment by seeing how many inches of flab you can pinch! (No warm-up needed for this!)

Try the following test when you begin the *No Sweat Fitness* plan and then repeat it in six weeks. If you were overfat to start with you should see the figures start to decrease.

Pinch the following body sites and record the scores using you own (honest!) judgement. If you don't trust yourself to be truthful, ask your partner or friend to give you a hand!

### RATING

5 = a massive handful of flesh
4 = a substantial roll of flesh
3 = more than an inch of flesh
2 = between half an inch and one inch of flesh
1 = less than half an inch of flesh
0 = hardly any flesh

| DATE | BODY SITE | SCORE 0–5 |
|------|-----------|-----------|

**WEEK 1**

    TOP OF FRONT OF ARMS

    TOP OF BACK OF ARMS

    STOMACH – JUST ABOVE HIPS

    BACK – BELOW SHOULDER BLADES

    INNER THIGH

    LOWER PART OF BOTTOM

    SIDE OF BOTTOM – JUST ABOVE HIP-BONE LEVEL

                               TOTAL =

| DATE | BODY SITE | SCORE 0–5 |
|------|-----------|-----------|

**WEEK 6**

    TOP OF FRONT OF ARMS

    TOP OF BACK OF ARMS

    STOMACH – JUST ABOVE HIPS

    BACK – BELOW SHOULDER BLADES

    INNER THIGH

    LOWER PART OF BOTTOM

    SIDE OF BOTTOM – JUST ABOVE HIP-BONE LEVEL

                               TOTAL =

| DATE | BODY SITE | SCORE 0–5 |
|------|-----------|-----------|

**WEEK 12**

    TOP OF FRONT OF ARMS

    TOP OF BACK OF ARMS

    STOMACH – JUST ABOVE HIPS

    BACK – BELOW SHOULDER BLADES

    INNER THIGH

    LOWER PART OF BOTTOM

    SIDE OF BOTTOM – JUST ABOVE HIP-BONE LEVEL

                               TOTAL =

If you have been following the *No Sweat Fitness* programme, you should see these fat figures start to decrease. If you want to burn up more fat, remember to do lots of low intensity aerobic exercise such as walking (see pp74–5).

## AEROBIC FITNESS

Time how long it takes you to walk (or jog) a mile. Remember to warm up first (see THE WALKING PROGRAMME). Record this time and see if you can improve it over six weeks. If you find it too difficult to cover a whole mile, do the same test but with a shorter distance (e.g. half a mile).

| DATE | DISTANCE | TIME |
| --- | --- | --- |
| WEEK 1 | 1 MILE | |
| WEEK 6 | 1 MILE | |
| WEEK 12 | 1 MILE | |

## MUSCULAR STRENGTH AND ENDURANCE

See how many good quality repetitions of the following you can do in 30 seconds. Warm up first by going for a short walk (5–6 minutes), walking up and down stairs or just dancing around to music.

### BOX PRESS-UP

Kneel on the floor with your hands on the ground in front of you in a 'box position'. Check that your shoulders are over your hands and your back is straight. Lower your chin to the ground, keeping your back straight. Now push up to the starting position, making sure you don't lock out – i.e. totally straighten – your elbows. Try to do the whole movement to the two-second count of 1 ... 2 ... Repeat as many times as possible in 30 seconds. Record your score on the following page.

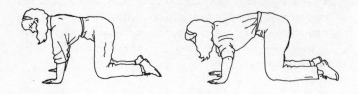

## CURL-UP

Lie on your back with your knees bent, feet flat on the floor and pelvis tucked in so that the small of your back is on the floor. Place your hands on your thighs. Curl up so that your fingers touch the top of your knees. Keep looking up and forward. If you feel a strain in the neck, concentrate on using your stomach muscles more, and

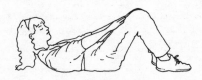

place one hand gently behind your head for support. Never forcibly yank your head forwards. Again try to do the whole movement to the two-second count of 1 ... 2 ... Repeat as many times as possible in 30 seconds. Record your score below.

| DATE | TEST | NUMBER OF REPS IN 30 SECONDS |
| --- | --- | --- |
| WEEK 1 | BOX-PRESS | |
| | CURL-UP | |
| WEEK 6 | BOX-PRESS | |
| | CURL-UP | |
| WEEK 12 | BOX-PRESS | |
| | CURL-UP | |

Don't worry if you find these exercises very strenuous at first. You can improve your muscular strength and endurance very quickly by following the guidelines and exercises in this book, and you should be able to do several more box-presses and curl-ups by Week 6, and even more by Week 12!

## FLEXIBILITY

Warm up first by going for a short walk (5–6 minutes) or just dancing around the house.

Place a box or crate next to a wall and tape a ruler on the top so that half of it sticks out over the edge. Now sit on the floor with your legs straight out in front of you and your feet flat against the box. Stretch forwards and measure how far you can reach with your finger tips.

| DATE | NUMBER OF INCHES |
| --- | --- |
| WEEK 1 | |
| WEEK 6 | |
| WEEK 12 | |

Remember, to improve your flexibility you really need to work at it every day, but for each of these four basic fitness tests you should be able to see a notable improvement over six weeks and even more after 12.

# TWENTY GOOD REASONS FOR
# GETTING FIT

To reduce your chance of coronary heart disease
To reduce your chance of osteoporosis
To slow down the ageing process
To reduce the chances of arthritis
To cope better under stress
To improve your circulation
To help your digestive system
To lose weight
To improve your posture
To be able to catch the bus
To walk up the Eiffel Tower
To be able to look down and see your feet
To have more energy to enjoy life
To be able to carry your own shopping home
To sleep better
To improve your skin tone
To feel more confident
To improve your sex life
To improve your balance
To improve your co-ordination

## SOME COMMON EXERCISE MYTHS

*'Swimming is one of the best ways to lose weight.'*
Swimming is an excellent exercise for improving your cardiovascular
fitness. It is also very safe for people who are overweight as their
body weight is supported. Swimming is not, however, a good way
to lose weight as fat is the body's natural buoyancy aid so swimming
encourages the storage of fat rather than the loss of it.

*'If I do weight-training I will end up with big, bulky muscles.'*
It is actually very hard to build up big muscles, even if you are male

and training regularly in a gym. Women are very unlikely to build up bulky muscles as they do not have enough testosterone, the hormone responsible for the development of muscle size.

*'If I do hundreds of leg-lifts every day, I'll soon have slim thighs.'*
It is impossible to reduce the size of one part of your body specifically. It is like saying that if you chew a lot of gum you will get a thin face! The body has a way of depositing fat in certain areas – which often means big bottoms and thighs for women, and stomachs and 'love handles' for men. The only way to reduce the size of these areas is to lose body fat all over. Unfortunately, you tend to lose the fat from places which are already quite slim, and bigger fat deposits take the longest to shed.

*'If I sit in a sauna for long enough, I'll lose weight.'*
If you weigh yourself directly after a sauna, the chances are you will be a couple of pounds lighter. But this is due to water loss and any 'weight' you have lost you will immediately put back on again when you have a drink. Saunas are not an effective way of losing weight. They are, however, very relaxing and can make you feel better at the end of a long, hard day.
      WARNING: Don't go into a sauna straight after exercising as this will prevent the body's natural cooling down period.

*'I'm very slim so I don't need to do any exercise.'*
Body weight is very misleading. You may be thin but you may have a high percentage of body fat, and if you do not do any exercise you may be very unfit. Alternatively, there are many 'fat' people who are very fit and healthy. If you are thin it is particularly important that you do some weight-bearing exercise to strengthen your bones (thin people are more prone to osteoporosis, or brittle-bone disease) and also aerobic exercise to strengthen your heart. The movements in this book will also help give your muscles more definition and so make you look more shapely.

*'When I stop exercising all my muscle will turn to fat.'*
Muscle and fat are two totally different things and they cannot be turned into each other. If you stop exercising you will lose muscle tone but this itself cannot turn into fat. If you stop exercising,

however, you will probably decrease your activity level so that you use up less energy and are therefore more likely to put on fat.

*'Squash is an excellent type of aerobic exercise.'*
For most people the game of squash involves a lot of stopping and starting. Unless you are very proficient you are unlikely to be able to sustain a 15–minute continuous rally which is the time needed to be of aerobic benefit. The level of intensity in playing squash is also very high which makes it anaerobic sometimes (without the presence of oxygen) and therefore dangerous for anyone suffering from high blood pressure or a weak heart.

'As you get older you need to slow down, put your feet up and not be so active.'

The older you get the more important it is to keep active and you have to put more effort into staying fit and healthy. Your body fat percentage increases with age so that, although you may weigh the same as you did ten years ago, you may actually be a lot fatter. You need to pay particular attention to mobility exercise to keep all your joints functioning properly. The risk of osteoporosis (brittle bone disease) also increases with age, particularly if you are female, although weight-bearing exercise (such as walking, cycling, jogging, badminton or tennis) will reduce this risk.

# PART THREE

## THE NO SWEAT WARM-UP AND COOL-DOWN

*REMEMBER! Part Three is part of your FITNESS TOOL-BOX. Don't skip it! You need to read this section carefully in order to be fully equipped to do the NO SWEAT FITNESS programme.*

Having read the SELF-ASSESSMENT section in Part Two, you will already know that you should be warmed up before doing any exercise or movements. The ones in this book are designed to be done at snatched moments throughout the day. Although you are not going to be exercising in a structured class environment, it is still important that you do a short warm-up before you start. If you do not, it is like trying to start a car in fifth gear. Your body will not be prepared.

In order to avoid injuries, you need to pay particular attention to preparing your joints for the work ahead. Imagine that they need oiling before they can move freely. Our natural joint lubricant is called synovial fluid, and mobility movements, like the ones below, will increase its flow, ensuring a greater range of movement and so reducing the chance of injury. Similarly, the warm-up will also increase the temperature in the deep muscles, preparing them for the work ahead so that your exercising will be more effective.

You do not have to do the whole NO SWEAT WARM-UP every time you want to do an exercise in this book. The amount of time you spend on it depends on several factors, such as room temperature, your personal fitness level and how long and intense your exercise session is going to be. If you can spend five to ten minutes warming up, that is excellent. If not, make sure you at least mobilise the area of the body you want to strengthen or stretch. All the exercises in this book include details of which body part they are designed to work. Use this as an indication as to which part of the body you need to mobilise. For example, if you want to do the Dirty Dishes Squat exercise on p93, designed to tone up the thighs and bottom, do some lower body mobility exercises such as Knee Bends and Hip Circles. Or if you are going to do the Shopper's Raise exercise on p107, designed to strengthen the shoulders, do some upper body mobility exercises such as Shoulder Rolls and Arm Circles – with a little practice, the NO SWEAT WARM-UP will become perfectly natural to you, and the movements are also excellent if you are feeling tense or sluggish. I like to do them as soon as I wake up to loosen up my joints which are stiff from sleeping, but they are also ideal if you have been sitting still for a long time at a desk or in front of the television.

Spend 10–30 seconds on each or any of the exercises below.

## LOWER BODY

### 1. ANKLE CIRCLES

For:  Mobilising the ankles
Coaching points:  Keep the neck and spine long
Reps:  5–15 clockwise
        5–15 anticlockwise

If you cannot balance on one leg, hold on to a wall or something for support. Stand with your feet hip-width apart, stomach pulled in and spine long. Bend your right knee slightly. Stretch your left leg out in front of you and slowly circle the ankle about half a dozen times in a clockwise direction and half a dozen times in an anti-clockwise direction. Repeat with the other leg.

This mobility exercise can also be done sitting at a desk, on a train or in an armchair in front of the television. It is a good way to promote circulation to the ankles and so prevent puffiness in this area.

### 2. HEEL RAISES

For:  Mobilising the ankles
Coaching points:  Walk through the whole foot
Reps:  5–15 on each foot

Stand tall, with your feet shoulder-width apart and toes pointing forwards. Now walk through your feet, rolling from the heel, through to the ball of the foot and then the toes. Try to make this a flowing, rhythmical movement and rise up on to the balls of your feet swinging your arms by your sides.

You can also do this warm-up exercise sitting on the edge of a chair, rolling through the feet.

## 3. KNEE BENDS

For: Mobilising the knees
Coaching points: Check that the knees stay over the toes
Don't squat too low

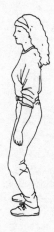

Stand tall, with your feet shoulder-width apart and knees slightly bent. Bend the knees further so that you lower your hips towards the floor. Then straighten them gently and return to the standing position. This should only be a small movement, not a full squat. Your knees should be over your toes, keeping the upper body tall.

## 4. KNEE RAISES

For: Mobilising the hips and knees
Coaching points: Keep the spine and neck long
Reps: 5–15 on each leg, alternating

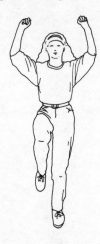

This is an excellent exercise to mobilise the hips and knees and is also good for raising the body temperature. Stand with your feet hip-width apart, toes pointing forwards, knees slightly bent. Raise your right knee straight up towards your chest, at the same time raising both arms up towards the ceiling. Lower the foot back to the floor, pulling back down with the arms. Repeat several times on alternate legs.

## 5. HIP CIRCLES

For: Mobilising the hips
Coaching points: Try not to move the upper body
Reps: 5–15 clockwise
        5–15 anticlockwise

Stand tall, feet shoulder-width apart and knees slightly bent. Place your hands on your hips and slowly circle them in a clockwise direction. Try to keep your upper body still and straight and isolate the movement from the hips. Change directions.

## UPPER BODY

### 6. SIDE BENDS

For:  Mobilising the sides of the body
Coaching points:  Do not lean forwards or backwards
                  Support your body weight with your hand on your
                  thigh
Reps:  5–15 each side

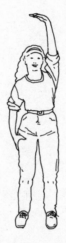

Stand tall, feet hip-width apart, knees slightly bent. Placing your right
hand on your right thigh, lift up and out of your hips towards the
ceiling with your left arm so that you feel a mild stretch down the
left side of your body. Concentrate on keeping your upper body
straight – imagine that there is a sheet of glass behind you and
another sheet in front of you so that you cannot lean backwards or
forwards. Return to the starting position, feeling that your spine is
being stretched up towards the ceiling. Repeat several times on each
side.

## 7. TORSO TWIST

For:  Mobilising the waist and torso
Coaching points:  Keep your hips pointing forwards
                  Keep your knees bent all the time
Reps:  5–15 each side

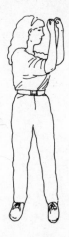

Stand tall, feet hip-width apart, knees slightly bent. Stretch your arms
out in front of you, then flex at the elbows so that your knuckles are
facing the ceiling and palms facing you. Now twist your torso to the
right, keeping the lower body fixed. Your hips should stay pointing
forwards. Return to the centre and repeat five times on each side.

## 8. SHOULDER ROLLS

For:  Mobilising the shoulders
Coaching points:  Keep your arms down and neck and spine long
Reps:  5–15 forwards
5–15 backwards

Stand tall, feet shoulder-width apart, knees slightly bent, resting your
finger-tips on the outside of your thighs. Roll your shoulders forwards
bringing them up towards your ears and then pressing them backwards in a big circle, keeping your arms relaxed, and finger-tips
resting on your thighs. Keep your neck and spine long. Repeat for
the desired number of reps and then change the direction of the roll.

## 9. ARM CIRCLES

For: Mobilising the shoulders
Coaching points: Keep the neck and spine long
Reach up to the ceiling with each circle
Keep the lower body still
Reps: 5–10 forwards
5–10 backwards

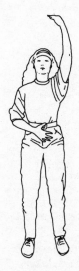

Stand tall, feet hip-width apart, knees slightly bent. Place your right palm on the centre of your stomach. Reach up to the ceiling with your left arm and circle it backwards for the desired number of reps. Repeat, circling it forwards. Try to keep the lower body still to isolate the movement in the shoulder. Repeat on the other side.

## 10. NECK ROLLS

For: Mobilising the neck
Coaching points: Keep the spine long
Do not roll the neck backwards
Reps: 5–10

Stand tall, feet shoulder-width apart, knees slightly bent. Keeping the rest of your body still, turn your head to the right. Now gently circle it forwards, through the centre and over to the left. Avoid tipping your head back as this is dangerous for the neck. Repeat for the desired number of reps.

## TEMPERATURE RAISERS

Your joints should now be fully mobilised and ready for ACTION. If it is very cold or you do not feel warmed up enough yet for further exercise, do one or more of the following temperature raisers.

### ARM RUNNING

Stand with your feet hip-width apart, spine and neck long, knees slightly bent. Bend your arms slightly and make a running motion with them, bringing one arm forward as you take the other arm back. Allow your knees to bend and straighten with the motion.

### STAIR CLIMBING

Do 'step ups' (excellent for toning the thighs and bottom) by standing at the bottom of the stairs and just stepping up on to the first stair and down. As you step up make sure that you are standing tall, that you land with the whole foot and that your toes are pointing forwards. Alternate the leading foot.

### DANCING

Put the radio or your favourite record on and just dance around the room.

### JOGGING ON THE SPOT

Jog on the spot – but if you are doing this for more than a few seconds make sure you are wearing appropriate jogging shoes. Keep the spine and neck long and check that your whole foot lands on the floor with each step. Keep the arms loose and relaxed.

## WALK IT OUT

Go for a five-minute walk outside or indoors (see THE WALKING PROGRAMME), swinging your arms to help increase your body temperature.

When you do aerobic exercise, you also need to prepare the cardiovascular system by raising the heart rate gradually. An easy way to do this is just to start the exercise at a very low intensity. For example, in THE WALKING PROGRAMME, you would walk at a slow pace for about five minutes, building up to a brisk walk gradually. Alternatively, you could spend five minutes doing THE TEMPERATURE RAISERS above. In this way there will not be such a shock to the circulatory and respiratory systems and you should not feel any discomfort. The fitter you get, the less time it will take you to warm up and get ready for action.

## THE COOL-DOWN

At the end of any strenuous work-out you also need to change down gears again. This is not so important if you have only been doing a few stretching or toning exercises, but if you have increased your heart rate considerably (e.g. with brisk walking) you should spend the last few minutes slowing the pace down and gradually getting your heart rate back to normal again. Never stop suddenly after any sort of aerobic exercise. This can make you feel faint and dizzy as the blood has not had time to circulate back from the working muscles to the brain, and you are also endangering your heart, because the blood pools down in your legs and cannot get back up to your heart which is still beating at an elevated rate. By cooling down gradually you also help the body get rid of substances such as lactic acid which build up in the working muscles and can cause stiffness and soreness later.

# PART FOUR

## THE NO SWEAT TECHNIQUE

*REMEMBER! Part Four is part of your FITNESS TOOL-BOX. Don't skip it! You need to read this section carefully in order to be fully equipped to do the NO SWEAT FITNESS programme.*

## CORRECT TECHNIQUE

The most essential part of *No Sweat Fitness* is not *what* you do but *how* you do it. After years of working out and writing about fitness, I am convinced that the way to change your body shape lies purely in correct technique.

I know many women who have been doing exercise classes for years and never improved their figure as they have been doing the exercises incorrectly. In fact, many of them end up with bigger, bulkier muscles than before. There is no point doing scores of leg lifts if you are not controlling the correct muscles. Indeed, by doing an exercise incorrectly you are also increasing the risk of injury. Alternatively, I know many people who have fantastic figures who have never done a leg lift or an organised exercise routine in their life! They are in good shape because they know how to carry themselves and always use their muscles to maximum effect, even if they are only picking up a piece of paper from the floor. Everything they do looks graceful and effortless instead of clumsy and laboured.

Many people who go to exercise classes think that as soon as they step out of the studio they can relax and stop using their bodies. But correct movement should be a part of everyday life, not something you set aside for so many minutes a day. You need to spend a few days concentrating on every little movement you make and trying to do everything with more deliberation and control. To move correctly you don't need to involve the whole body – you can focus on the specific muscle required for that particular task while keeping the rest of the body relaxed and tension free. When you do a leg lift, for example, you should concentrate on moving only the leg while the upper body stays still, and once you start developing this sense of body awareness you will quickly see an improvement in your shape and overall appearance.

Every exercise in this book includes details of which muscles it is designed to work so you can concentrate specifically on this particular area. Make sure you follow all the instructions carefully. I have included coaching tips to ensure that all the movements are as safe and effective as possible. You will find that nearly all the exercises, including those in the warm-up section, involve pulling in your stomach and keeping your neck and spine long. Not only will this help improve your posture and prevent injury, but it also means that you will end up with a beautifully toned stomach without having to do specific abdominal exercises. So remember – keep that tummy pulled in!    •

Try to perfect one movement at a time. It is better to learn just a few exercises properly than trying to do too many and ending up with poor technique. Take your time. Remember – this is fitness for life so it does not matter if you learn only a couple of exercises a week.


# CONTRAINDICATIONS AND RULES

*No Sweat Fitness* is a very safe and carefully devised exercise programme. Make sure you have read the SELF-ASSESSMENT safety points and stop exercising and consult your GP immediately if any of the following happens:

1. extreme difficulty in breathing;
2. dizziness;
3. nausea or vomiting;
4. irregular heart rate after exercise;
5. loss of co-ordination;

   6. tightness in chest or pain related to teeth, arm, jaw, ear or
      upper back.
Finally, do not exercise if:
   1. you have a cold or flu;
   2. you have eaten or been drinking alcohol in the last hour or
      two;
   3. you have an injury and have not had permission to use this
      programme from your specialist.

# POSTURE

Another vital ingredient of *No Sweat Fitness* is good posture. If you
are incorrectly aligned you will not be able to move efficiently.

Good posture is something you need to be aware of 24 hours
a day whether you are sitting at a desk, gardening or lifting the baby
out of the bath. I suggest you spend a couple of weeks concentrating
on this and you will be amazed how much your whole body lifts,
your stomach flattens and your appearance improves once you are
correctly aligned.

Try the following test to see if your body is correctly aligned.
Before you can improve your posture you need to be aware of where
it goes wrong.

## POSTURE TEST

If you don't have good posture you will find the first position
exhausting. Don't worry – it will get easier as your posture improves
from doing the exercises in this section. Do this test three times a
week for a couple of weeks and record the results on the table below.
It will help realign your body and lift and strengthen your stomach
muscles.

## 11. THE POSTURE TEST

Stand with your heels about two inches from a wall, feet hip-width
apart. You should not be touching the wall yet at all. Now slowly
press your body backwards, with your toes still touching the ground.

If you have good posture just your hair, shoulder-blades and bottom should touch the wall. If you feel that one side of your body touches before the other, you are lop-sided. There should only be a small gap between your lower back and the wall – if you can place a whole fist there or your shoulders touch the wall before your bottom, your pelvis is too far forward and you need to practise The Pelvic Tilt (see below).

Assess yourself from the categories below. You may find that you record a combination of points to start with. Continue this test for longer if you have not started to score one consistently after the first two weeks. This is a good test to use once a month as a check-up.

1 = perfect alignment (hair, shoulder-blades and bottom touching the wall; ear, shoulder, hip and knee should all be aligned)

2 = pelvis too far forward (shoulders touch wall before bottom; big gap between lower back and wall). Keep practising the Pelvic Tilt below

3 = tense neck (neck is curved inwards, with tight, tensed-up muscles). Practise lengthening the neck by Standing Tall (see below)

4 = sway-backed knees (calves touch wall). If you have overextended knees, make sure you don't snap them back and always keep them very marginally bent)

5 = shoulders hunched (bottom touches wall before shoulders). Neck needs to be lengthened (see Stand Tall below)

6 = lop-sided (right side touches wall before left)

7 = lop-sided (left side touches wall before right)

| WEEK 1 | WEEK 2 |
| --- | --- |
| 1. | |
| 2. | |
| 3. | |

Many of the movements in this book will help improve your posture, but always read the instructions carefully and concentrate on the way you perform the movement. Strong muscles, particularly in the back and stomach, will help give you good carriage and support your spine. In this section, though, I have included a series of simple movements specifically designed to improve your posture and help back pain. These take hardly any time to do and can easily be incorporated into an everyday routine.

## 12. PELVIC TILTS

Coaching points: Keep the buttocks relaxed
Reps: 1–2

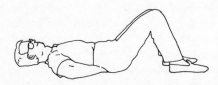

Lie on your back with your knees bent at 45 degrees and feet flat on the floor. Put one hand under the small of your back and feel the gap between that and the floor. Now press the small of your back into the floor and your hand by tightening your stomach muscles. Keep your buttock muscles relaxed and your neck long.

Now try the pelvic tilt standing against a wall, as in the Posture Test above. Bend your knees slightly, keeping both heels on the floor and feel your lower back press against the wall. Now straighten your knees and tighten your stomach muscles so that the pelvis rotates backwards and you flatten the space between your lower back and the wall. Remember to keep your buttock muscles relaxed and neck long.

## 13. STAND TALL

For: Lengthening the neck and spinal column
Coaching points: Keep your shoulders relaxed
Reps: 1–2

It is very important when doing any of the movements in this book to have a long neck that is devoid of tension. To get the feeling of a long neck, stand feet hip-width apart, stomach pulled in and pelvis slightly tilted (as in The Pelvic Tilt above). Now, keeping your head upright and chin pointing down towards the floor, lengthen your neck. Imagine that someone is pulling you up from above with a piece of string. Keep your shoulders relaxed and chest open. Be conscious of your feet being placed firmly on the ground and a force that is stretching your whole body and neck upwards.

NB: *Think of this position whenever you are reminded to 'stand tall' in this book.*

## SWEEPING THE FLOOR

Use sweeping the floor as an excuse to work on your posture! The following movement will improve posture and streamline your waist, and can be done holding the handle of a broom or mop or with an imaginary long stick.

## 14. THE STRAIGHT SWEEP

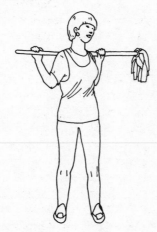

For:  Improving the posture
        Trimming the waist
Coaching point:  Keep the lower body still
Reps:  5–10 each side

Stand tall, knees bent, feet hip-width apart and toes pointing forward. Stretch your arms out sideways, holding a long stick across your shoulders. Pull in your stomach and gently swing from side to side from the waist, keeping your hips square and still. Repeat 5–10 times each side.

The simple and pleasurable movement that follows will strengthen and stretch both the back and the abdominal muscles.

## 15. CAT'S BACK

Coaching points:  Move smoothly – NEVER jerk
                  Keep your neck lengthened
Reps: 5–10

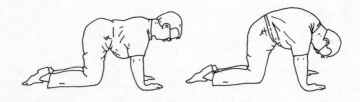

Kneel on all fours with your hands and knees about shoulder-width apart. Drop your stomach and chest towards the floor while raising your bottom towards the ceiling. Keep your neck lengthened. Now drop your head and arch your back upwards. Repeat 5–10 times.

### THE BACK

People often make the mistake of strengthening their stomach muscles while neglecting the muscles in their back. This can lead to postural imbalance and potential back problems. Do this back strengthening movement when you are lying in front of the television, last thing at night or whenever you have a spare moment.

## 16. THE BEACHED WHALE

Coaching points:  Spend the same amount of time going down as
                  lifting up again
                  Keep the neck and spine lengthened
Reps:  5–15

Lie face down on the floor with the backs of your hands resting on
your bottom. Now slowly raise your head and chest a few inches

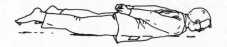

above the ground. Keep your neck lengthened. This is a very subtle
movement and there should be no feeling of straining. Slowly lower
your chest and head back towards the ground but do not touch the
floor. Never crash down – spend the same effort lowering yourself
as raising yourself. Lower and lift 5–15 times.

## WALL WINNERS

The following movements are excellent for improving your posture.
Do them whenever you have a spare moment and are near some
wall space, such as when you are in the kitchen waiting for the kettle
to boil or in between batches of work at the office.

## 17. WALL WINNER I

Coaching points:  Keep your spine and neck lengthened
Reps:  2–3

Stand with your back to the wall, heels 2–3 inches away from it and
knees slightly bent. You should only be touching the wall lightly with
your hair, shoulder-blades and bottom. Do the pelvic tilt. Stretch
spine up and along wall and keep lengthening your neck and spine
all the time, your arms in front of your body and fingers lightly
touching. Now stretch your arms out sideways so that you trace a
big graceful circle with your hands, ending up with your arms
stretched up above your head, fingers lightly touching. Make sure
you don't sink down the wall, arch your back or hunch your shoulders.

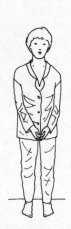
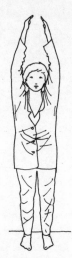

Try to stretch your head higher as your arms are raised. Lower your arms back to the starting position, maintaining this feeling of stretch in the arms and body and keeping your neck and spine long. Repeat 2–3 times.

## 18. WALL WINNER II

Coaching points:  As for Ex 17
Reps:  1

Stand with your heels against the wall and knees slightly bent, with only your hair, shoulder-blades and bottom lightly touching the wall. Close your eyes for five seconds and imagine that you have a set of springs in all your joints so that when you walk away you will feel light and sprightly!

## BEDTIME SOOTHERS

Shoulders and backs are particularly tense at the end of the day. Make the following soothing movements part of your bedtime routine – they don't take any longer than brushing your teeth or cleaning your face and will make you have a much better and more comfortable night's sleep.

## 19. BEDTIME SPACE

Coaching point: Keep your hips forward
Reps: 2–3 each side

Stand in front of a mirror, with your knees bent and fingers gently touching in front of you to create a space of air between your arms

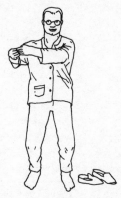

and body. Keeping this same 'space', turn to the right from your waist to look over your right shoulder. Your hips should remain square and pointing forwards. Keep your shoulders back and head high. Repeat on the other side, always keeping the same 'space' between your arms and body. This should feel as though you're being massaged between the shoulder-blades. Repeat 2–3 times on each side.

## 20. BEDTIME STAR

For: Stretching out the lower back
Coaching points: Keep your stomach pulled in
              Keep your knees tightly pressed together
Hold: 10–20 seconds each side

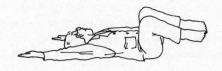

Lie on your back in a star position with your arms stretched out above your head. Bring your knees up to your chest. Pull in your stomach and roll your knees to the right side of your body. At the same time turn your head to the left and stretch out your left arm. Hold for 10–20 seconds, and repeat on the other side.

## GENERAL EVERYDAY POSTURE TIPS

1. Be aware of your body alignment at all times. When you are correctly aligned, the body is at its most efficient and there is a sensation of lightness and freedom.

2. Avoid any kind of movement or exercise that involves a rounded back. When the back is rounded there is more stress on the spinal structure and an increased risk of slipping a disc. The golden rule is always to bend at the knees while keeping your back straight and head up. Avoid sitting in something like a hammock or deck chair which encourages a rounded spine.

3. Always squat or kneel instead of bending over when weeding, hoeing or planting in the garden.

4. When lifting a heavy box or crate keep it as close to your body as possible and keep your feet hip-width apart with one foot slightly in front of the other to create a stable base. Use your leg muscles as the main source of power rather than relying on your back. Remember to keep your legs bent but back straight. Use the pelvic tilt.

5. Never try to lift something that is too heavy for you.

6. When you are lifting a heavy load, ask someone to help you or else, if possible, break it up into smaller parcels.

7. Don't sit with your legs crossed. This can cause curvature of the spine and stresses the spinal structure.

8. Avoid wearing high heels as this will push your body out of alignment.

9. When driving a car, try to keep your head and shoulders relaxed. Don't lock your head back on to your neck or hunch your

shoulders. If the seat does not come up right to the top of your head, add a neck support.

10. Don't hunch your back when washing-up or preparing vegetables. Try placing the bowl on top of the draining board so you don't have to stoop. When ironing, adjust the board to waist height.

11. If you are a typist or someone who has to keep looking at something to one side, try and vary which side of the typewriter you keep the work on. You do not want to strain your neck by having to keep twisting to the same side.

12. Try not to carry heavy shopping or suitcases on one particular side all the time. Alternate the hand you carry them with.

13. If you carry a baby in a sling, have it on your back like a rucksack rather than strapped to your chest. Choose a cot that is a comfortable height so you don't have to keep stooping over to pick up the child.

14. When making the bed or cleaning the bath, avoid stooping by doing it in a kneeling position.

15. When hanging out the washing, bring the line down to a comfortable level so you don't have to reach up too high.

16. If you have to stand up all day at work, try to keep moving and shifting your weight. Stand on tip-toes, bend your knees and tense and relax different muscle groups such as the bottom, stomach and thighs.

17. If possible, pull rather than push a heavy object, as this will put less stress on your lower back.

18. Be particularly careful about your back first thing in the morning as you won't be at your most co-ordinated and your discs are vulnerable.

# BREATHING

Correct breathing is another vital component of *No Sweat Fitness*. Breathing properly will improve your circulation and digestion, make you feel more comfortable and relaxed, strengthen the stomach muscles and help protect the back from injury.

Most people breathe using their ribs and upper chest, but the correct way to breathe is actually lower down, using the diaphragm and stomach muscles. If you use your ribs all the time for breathing, the muscles here will become very tight and exhausted.

Many people who exercise make the mistake of sucking in their breath when they lift a weight or do anything strenuous. It is actually much easier and more effective if you breathe *out* on exertion as this will relax the muscles so they can stretch or strengthen that little bit more. Stomach exercises are a classic example of when people try to hold their breath. If you breathe out as you pull in your stomach muscles, you will get a much better result as the muscles will lengthen and look flat rather than bunched up. Try to incorporate this correct breathing pattern into everyday life, so that, for example, you breathe out with the exertion of lifting up a heavy object or when rising from a chair.

The following movement is very simple and will teach you how to breathe using your stomach muscles.

## 21. BLOW UP THE BALLOON

Coaching point:  Spend some time inhaling and exhaling
Reps:  5–15

Lie on your back with your knees bent at 45 degrees and feet flat on the floor. Keep your neck long and chest and upper ribs relaxed. Place both palms on your stomach. Concentrate on feeling your stomach move as you breathe. Now imagine that there is a balloon inside your stomach that slowly fills up with air as you breathe in and then slowly deflates as you breathe out. Try and make the cycle of breathing very smooth and regular so that it takes the same time to blow the balloon up as it does to deflate it.

Once you are used to the breathing exercise above you can do the following movement in a standing position, whenever you have a spare moment – at a bus stop, in the supermarket queue or on the tube.

## 22. STAND AND BREATHE

Coaching point:  Keep your spine and neck lengthened
Reps:  5–10

Stand tall, feet hip-width apart, knees slightly bent, hands on hips. Breathe in slowly feeling your stomach expand. Breathe out, sucking in your stomach so it presses flat against your back. Relax (keeping your shoulders down). Repeat 5–10 times. Keep your spine and neck lengthened throughout.

Finally, try the following exercise (derived from the Alexander Technique) to help loosen the jaw and expand the rib-cage.

## 23. OPEN MOUTHED

Coaching points:  Keep your shoulders relaxed
Reps:  2–3

Stand tall, feet hip-width apart, knees slightly bent, hands on hips. Breathe in slowly feeling your stomach expand. This time as you breathe out open your mouth and let the soft sound of 'AH!' come out. Repeat slowly 3–5 times.

WELL DONE! You have now completed the crucial Part Four of the *No Sweat Fitness* plan. Re-read this section whenever possible. I still do many of the movements from this section on a regular basis and the more you can improve your technique, posture and breathing, the nearer you are to achieving *No Sweat Fitness* for life!

# PART FIVE

## THE WALKING PROGRAMME

*REMEMBER! Part Five is part of your FITNESS TOOL-BOX. Don't skip it! It is a very important section in the NO SWEAT FITNESS programme and the key to your aerobic fitness.*

Walking is the most natural and easy way to keep fit. It is the ultimate *No Sweat* activity as it is so simple to incorporate into everyday life and it plays a very important part in the *No Sweat Fitness* programme as it will get you aerobically fit, boost your metabolic rate and relax your mind.

In the Caucuses, where people live well into their hundreds, walking really is a way of life. After autopsy, it was discovered that many of them had actually had heart attacks earlier in life and not noticed as they were so aerobically fit.

Walking, like running or cycling, is an aerobic exercise as it improves the function of your heart and lungs. It is also a low-impact exercise so it puts minimal stress on joints and muscles and is therefore safer than a high-impact exercise such as running. From the body beautiful point of view, walking is also an excellent way to burn fat – burning about 200 calories in half an hour. Walk uphill and you increase this by another 100 calories, and walking downhill actually takes even more effort as you have to brake.

If you are trying to lose weight it is better to do long periods of brisk walking than short bursts of running, because the body burns more fat when it is working at a low intensity for long periods of time. To lose one pound of fat you have to burn up on average about 3,500 calories. That equates to having to walk about 35 miles – a long way to go just to get rid of one pound of fat! But before you pack away your walking shoes, don't despair! If you were just to walk a mile a day briskly for a year, you would burn up the equivalent of over ten pounds in body fat, without having to diet or cut back on your calorie intake.

*No Sweat Fitness* works by increasing your metabolic rate rather than calorie counting. By going for a walk, your metabolic rate will actually be increased for up to 24 hours after you have come back, so walking has an accumulative effect – the more you do, the more you will keep your metabolic rate charged and the more fat you will burn. If you do want to lose weight, try to walk for as long as possible, preferably for 20–30 minutes four or five times a week. To get an aerobic effect you need to do at least 15 minutes continuous brisk walking two or three times a week. Remember – you need to walk fast enough to feel warm and slightly breathless, but not so fast that you can not comfortably hold a conversation. The important thing, however, is to make walking a part of your everyday life. Don't think upon it as 'exercise' or a 'chore'. Walking can be so enjoyable. It enables you to get out in the fresh air, to have time on your own to do some constructive thinking, to unwind or to chat with a friend.

Walking is principally a lower-body activity, excellent for toning legs and buttocks, while swinging the arms will help work the shoulders and arms. The most important thing to remember is to WALK FAST. Even if you are just going a couple of hundred yards to your local shops, try and walk at a good pace. Keep your weight slightly forward and push off from the heels and through the toes as you go. Swing your arms like a pendulum. Try to create a sensation of energy, and stride out. This will help condition the thighs and bottom and make you feel alert and energised. On longer walks, try to cover a mile in 15 minutes.

Think how you could incorporate more walking into everyday life. If you live within a mile or two from work, you could easily walk it. If you drive to work, try to park the car further away than usual and walk the last 15 minutes. Or why not get off the tube or bus one stop early and walk the rest? As I work from home, I know how easy it is to be sedentary all day. When I first stopped working in an office, I was horrified to discover that I put on nearly a stone in weight in six months – simply because my activity level had dropped so drastically. Whereas previously I used to rush to work in the morning and virtually sprint half a mile to the local station, I was now walking only a few yards from my bedroom to my desk. I became so inactive that I had no energy, missing fresh air and having to have a nap almost every afternoon to keep myself going. It became a big expedition just to go round the corner and buy a pint of milk.

So, be warned! If your life is based in the home, you need to pay particular attention to increasing your activity and energy levels. Force yourself to go for a brisk 15–30-minute walk every lunchtime, and you'll be surprised how much more alert and refreshed it will make you feel. Use your daily walk as a way of doing something constructive. Walk a mile further to a shop that you do not usually bother visiting; walk round to see your friend rather than taking the car; and walk to the main post office rather than just popping a letter through the nearest post-box. At weekends, why not make walking in the countryside or along the city canals a way of spending time with your partner, friends or family? And if you really want to increase the fitness benefits, try hill-walking or even going on a special walking holiday.

## WALKING TIPS

1. Wear sturdy comfortable shoes.

2. Use the whole of the foot and push off firmly from the back leg.

3. Walk tall. Concentrate on keeping your spine and neck lengthened and stomach pulled in.

4. Walk at a brisk pace. For an aerobic effect, walk continuously for a minimum of 15 minutes, two or three times a week. To burn fat try to walk for 20–30 minutes, four or five times a week. Remember – to burn fat, walk fast enough to feel slightly breathless.

5. Always try to tell your family or friends where you are going for a walk and when you will be back.

6. Find as many opportunities as possible to go for a walk. It may be feasible to take a 15-minute walk instead of a coffee break. Alternatively, if you are going out for a business lunch, choose

a restaurant that is about 15 minutes' walk from your office so that you can walk there and back.

7. Go for a walk with your partner after dinner. This will give you time to chat without the distraction of television or the telephone ringing, help digest your food and get your metabolic rate going.

8. Walking can be romantic! Instead of going out for a dinner date, why not have a candlelit meal at home and afterwards go for a long romantic walk hand in hand.

9. Find a regular time of day that suits you to walk. It does not matter if this is early in the morning, part of your coffee break, lunchtime or an evening stroll. For *No Sweat Fitness* to work, you have to make walking part of your routine.

10. Buy a pedometer, a small device that hooks on to your belt and tells you how far you have walked. Before you start you have to programme it with your personal stride length. This will also help motivate you as you can time how long it takes you to walk a mile.

11. Follow the FIVE EASY STEPS TO WALKING below.


# FIVE EASY STEPS TO WALKING

Follow the five steps below to make your walking programme safe and effective.

## STEP ONE

Remember the principles of the NO SWEAT WARM-UP? If not, re-read them again now! The simplest way to warm up for brisk walking is to start with five minutes walking at a slow pace, swinging your arms to help raise your body temperature. As you get fitter you may find you do not need to spend more than a couple of minutes warming up.

## STEP TWO

Now that your muscles are nice and warm, spend a further minute or two doing some gentle stretching in preparation for the brisk walk ahead. You want to keep your body as still as possible when you stretch – trees, walls, lamp-posts and park-benches are all good obstacles to hold on to for support. Before brisk walking, hold each stretch for 6–10 seconds on each side. Don't push these stretches too hard as they are just part of the warm-up.

### 24. CALF STRETCH

Coaching point: Keep your toes pointing forwards
Hold: 6–10 seconds each side (Step Two)
        15–30 seconds each side (Step Five)

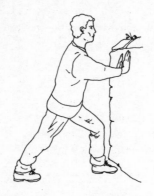

Stand facing a wall or tree for support, feet shoulder-width apart. Step forwards with one leg so that your back leg is straight and front leg is bent. Check that the toes of both feet are pointing forwards. Tilt your pelvis so that you feel a mild stretch down the calf of the back leg. Repeat on the other leg.

### 25. LOWER CALF STRETCH

Coaching point: Keep toes pointing forwards
Hold: 6–10 seconds each side (Step Two)
        15–30 seconds each side (Step Five)

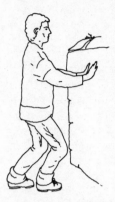

Stand, as for the Calf Stretch above. This time, slide your back foot forwards so that it is about six inches behind the front foot. Transfer your weight on to the back foot and, with both legs bent, sit back on to your back foot. This stretches out the lower part of the calf. Change legs.

## 26. HAMSTRING STRETCH

Coaching points:  Keep your neck and spine long and head up
                          Keep your supporting leg facing the bench
Hold:  6–10 seconds on each leg (Step Two)
          15–30 seconds on each leg (Step Five)

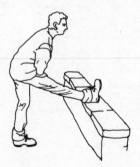

Stand, feet hip-width apart facing a park-bench or low wall with your hands on your thigh for balance, place your right foot on the bench and lean forwards from the waist until you feel a stretch in the back of the raised leg. Hold for the desired number of seconds. Change legs.

## 27. THIGH STRETCH

Coaching point:  Check that your knee is pointing directly down to
                        the floor
Hold:  6–10 seconds each side (Step Two)
          15–30 seconds each side (Step Five)

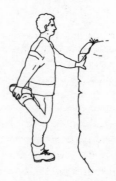

Hold on to a tree with your left hand for support. Hold your right foot with your right hand so that you pull your right heel towards your bottom. Check that the right knee is pointing towards the floor and that both are quite close together. Tilt your pelvis forwards slightly and you should feel a mild stretch down the front of your right thigh. Repeat on the other side.

## 28. REACH FOR THE SKY

Coaching point:  Avoid leaning backwards or forwards
Hold:  6–10 seconds each side (Step Two)
          (Not applicable for Step Five)

Stand feet hip-width apart, toes pointing forwards, bending the knees slightly and tipping the pelvis forwards. Place your left hand on your left thigh. Now stretch up towards the sky with your right arm so

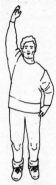

that you feel a mild stretch down the right side of the body. Keep your stomach pulled in and spine long. Repeat on the other side.

## 29. STOMACH STREAMLINER

Now that you have warmed up and done some preparatory stretching for your brisk walk, spend a minute or two concentrating on your stomach muscles. As you walk, be aware of your breathing. Every time you breathe out, contract your stomach muscles in. Stand up as tall as possible, keep your shoulders down and feel your stomach muscles pull back and lengthen. Relax your stomach as you breathe in but make sure your spine and neck stay long.

This simple exercise can be done at any time – walking, standing or sitting still – and is very effective for toning up the tummy muscles. With practice, you will be able to do it when walking briskly or even jogging. Remember – the more you practise it, the more streamlined your stomach will become!

## STEP THREE

Gradually increase the pace of your walking until you feel comfortably breathless. Continue at this pace for 15 minutes or more (see THE WALKING PROGRAMME below).

## STEP FOUR

Spend the last three to five minutes slowing the pace down. Keep your arms above your head if you feel faint or light-headed as this will keep your blood circulating to your heart and head.

## STEP FIVE

Finally, spend another couple of minutes doing some stretching to help develop your flexibility. Repeat stretches 24 to 27, this time pushing up yourself a little harder and holding up each stretch for 15–30 seconds.

*This five-step walking plan can be completed in under 30 minutes. Please don't skip any of the steps as they are important for making this programme safe and effective.*

# THE WALKING PROGRAMME

You should already have increased the amount of walking you do having read the ENERGY section. Now start concentrating on walking faster and longer distances and monitoring your results on the charts below. Remember – to strengthen your heart and lungs you need to do at least 15 minutes of brisk walking two or three times per week. If you are trying to lose weight aim to do 20–30 minutes of brisk walking four to five times per week.

As you get fitter you can increase the amount of walking you do. Remember – you need to walk fast enough to make yourself feel slightly breathless so that as you get fitter you will have to increase your speed to obtain this effect. It is also a good idea for the first few weeks to record what time of day you do your walk, enabling you to see a pattern emerging of the most convenient times for you to incorporate walking into your schedule. You may find, for example, that lunchtimes are most convenient for you so that you can make a lunchtime walk a regular part of your life.

If you use the charts below for four weeks, you should find that you can walk further in the allotted time. Measure the distance you walk with a pedometer, or, if you don't have one, use a route for which you know the exact distance (e.g. perhaps you have measured this in your car).

Again, award yourself points out of five as to how much you feel you have exerted yourself on each walk. For maximum *No Sweat Fitness* benefits, keep increasing the length and intensity of your walking weeks – I always try to walk for at least 30 minutes every day during the week and about an hour at weekends. You may also find it useful to make a copy of the charts below and pin them on to your front door as a reminder to go out and walk yourself thin!

TOD = time of day you went walking (e.g. 1.30–1.50 p.m.)
DURATION = time spent walking
DISTANCE = distance walked
E = exertion rate. Aim for a minimum total of 16 in the E column
    each week. Over 20 is excellent

    5 = flat out or brisk uphill
    4 = brisk
    3 = good steady pace
    2 = stroll
    1 = stop and start (e.g. window shopping)
    0 = stayed at home

## WEEK 1

| DAY | TOD | DURATION | DISTANCE | E |
|-----|-----|----------|----------|---|
| MON | | | | |
| TUE | | | | |
| WED | | | | |
| THUR | | | | |
| FRI | | | | |
| SAT | | | | |
| SUN | | | | |
| **TOTAL** | | | | |

## WEEK 2

Follow the *No Sweat Fitness* principle of progression. Try to walk faster this week so that you increase the distance you walk and the exertion rate.

| DAY | TOD | DURATION | DISTANCE | E |
|------|-----|----------|----------|---|
| MON | | | | |
| TUE | | | | |
| WED | | | | |
| THUR | | | | |
| FRI | | | | |
| SAT | | | | |
| SUN | | | | |
| **TOTAL** | | | | |

## WEEK 3

Follow the *No Sweat Fitness* principle of progression. Try to go for some longer walks this week. By now you should be spending at least 20 minutes on each walk so if you are trying to lose weight, go for one blow-out walk at the weekend (30 minutes plus), and make sure your exertion rates are the same, if not higher than in Week 2.

| DAY | TOD | DURATION | DISTANCE | E |
|------|-----|----------|----------|---|
| MON | | | | |
| TUE | | | | |
| WED | | | | |
| THUR | | | | |
| FRI | | | | |
| SAT | | | | |
| SUN | | | | |
| **TOTAL** | | | | |

## WEEK 4

Remember the *No Sweat Fitness* principle of progression. Make sure your exertion rate stays high and increase the distance and time you spend walking. Try to walk for 30 minutes on several days and again, if you are trying to lose weight, go for one long blow-out walk of 40 minutes. Keep going – you are doing well!

| DAY | TOD | DURATION | DISTANCE | E |
|---|---|---|---|---|
| MON | | | | |
| TUE | | | | |
| WED | | | | |
| THUR | | | | |
| FRI | | | | |
| SAT | | | | |
| SUN | | | | |
| TOTAL | | | | |

## JOGGING – NATURAL PROGRESSION

You will quickly feel the benefits of this walking programme. You will feel more energetic, alert and agile, your muscles will feel tighter and firmer, you will get less breathless when running up stairs and doing everyday tasks, your skin tone should improve through better circulation and you should also be sleeping much more soundly. It is a myth that exercise increases your appetite. For most people it is actually the reverse and all this extra walking should have decreased your appetite and made you feel like eating healthier foods (see FOOD FOR HEALTH).

However, once you start getting fitter, you may be inspired to take it further and do other aerobic exercise. You could, for example, substitute some of the walking sessions for swimming or cycling (see NO SWEAT SPORT for details of these sports), but you must always remember the *No Sweat* principle of progression. Keep thinking of ways of increasing your activity level further, for if you have been walking for weeks, you may find your heart gets so fit that, however fast you walk, you don't feel breathless any more. Unfortunately, when you are fit, you can actually 'lose' your fitness by exercising at too low an intensity.

Although I always hated running at school, I became interested in jogging through doing this walking programme. A slow jog is the natural progression from all this brisk walking. Don't make it a chore. It really can be enjoyable, particularly if you go out into the park on a sunny day. Go for your walk as usual, but this time wearing a tracksuit and pair of running shoes. Warm up with about 5–10 minutes of brisk walking. Then do the walking stretches in the previous section for your calves, thighs and hamstrings and continue walking briskly for a couple of minutes. When you feel ready for it, start jogging very slowly. In fact, you may not actually be travelling any faster than when you were walking briskly, but when you start feeling tired or uncomfortably breathless, return to walking, and keep alternating this walking and jogging so that you feel comfortable throughout.

Now that you have improved your cardiovascular fitness, this will be much easier than you ever imagined. The first time I actually broke into a jog, I was amazed that I continued for 25 minutes without it being any effort. The reason was that I had done so much brisk walking that a slow jog was an easy progression. You will find that jogging gives you a different physical sensation and mental high. There are some days when I feel like walking (usually when I feel a need to slow down or when I have a lot to think about), and other days when I feel the need to push myself a little harder. Jogging can be very meditative. But for *No Sweat Fitness* it really does not matter if you walk or jog – just do what you enjoy and experiment to find what suits you best and keeps you comfortably breathless.

For more information about the benefits of jogging, see p170.

# FITNESS FOR
# LIFE

# THE HOME WORK-OUT

If you spend most of your time indoors at home, you probably find it particularly hard to motivate yourself to do physical exercise. As I've worked from home for years, I know how easy it is to sit around all day snacking as if you were going into hibernation, and when I first started working from home there were some days when I didn't even walk more than about ten metres. If you are confined to a small space such as a flat or house, you will really benefit from following this section of the *No Sweat Fitness* programme.

The movements in this section will be particularly useful for anyone who spends a lot of time in the house, whether you are a housewife, househusband, mother, nanny, au-pair, pensioner or one of the many people who now work from home such as a freelance journalist, designer, writer, computer analyst or accountant. But as we all spend part of our life at home doing boring household chores, this section is also suitable for everyone on the *No Sweat Fitness* programme.

As you will see, there are numerous opportunities to move about more in the home. Why not tone up while waiting for the kettle to boil or while making the bed? And watching television, soaking in the bath and even sitting on the toilet are also prime *No Sweat Fitness* moments. I have suggested everyday situations which are appropriate for doing exercises in the house, but feel free to do any of them during an odd moment which is appropriate for you. A couple of minutes' movement here and there throughout the day can be just as beneficial as a full-blown work-out. The secret is to make these movements part of your daily ritual so that they become as natural as brushing your teeth or combing your hair. Remember the *No Sweat Fitness* technique of concentrating on good posture, with a long neck and spine and your stomach pulled in, and this too will become second nature – whether exercising or not – ensuring a beautifully toned stomach. So once you have read this section there should be no excuse for you to sit around hibernating ever again!

# HOME TIPS

1. Make sure you have read Parts One to Five.

2. Always remember to spend a few minutes doing the NO SWEAT WARM-UP (see Part Three). One of the simplest ways to warm up in a house is just to walk around for a few minutes doing something specific such as shutting all the doors, opening all the windows or tidying up.

3. Remember that 'quality' is the key to *No Sweat Fitness*, so follow all the instructions very carefully and concentrate hard on what you are doing.

4. Remember the principle of progression. Build up the number of repetitions of each exercise gradually.

5. Try to put as much physical effort into everyday tasks as you can. For example, make a point of jumping up from the sofa to switch TV channels rather than using the remote control; wring out your clothes by hand rather than using the tumble-drier; get out of bed early at the weekend to wash the car yourself rather than taking it to the car-wash; empty the rubbish more often than usual; and do the gardening yourself.

6. If you live in a house, try to use the stairs as much as possible. Running up and down stairs is a great way to burn up calories and tone up the legs and bottom. To increase the strengthening effect, climb up two steps at a time.

7. Never sit still for more than an hour at a time. Get up and do any of the movements in this part as often as possible!

8. Wear loose, comfortable clothing when you are in the house so you are ready to do the stretches listed.

9. Use any opportunity to get outside and be as active as possible. For example, walk to the supermarket or video shop instead of driving, take the dog for a walk *before* he pesters you, and walk round to say hello to your neighbourhood friends instead of phoning.

10. Carrying shopping is a good way to tone up. In order to avoid back problems, make sure you distribute the load evenly so you have a bag in each hand. Even better, use a rucksack so that you take the weight on your back.

11. *No Sweat Fitness* starts the minute you wake up! Try to think ACTIVE as soon as you step out of bed and spend the first ten minutes of each day paying particular attention to everything you do, be it brushing your teeth or scrubbing yourself clean in the shower.

# THE HOUSEWORK-OUT

Not many of us actually like doing the housework, but it is, in fact, an excellent opportunity to tone up. Making the bed, for example, is a prime chance to tone up flabby thighs while hoovering is a good time to stretch out your calves. So put on that pinny and get beautifully toned while making your home look spruce and clean! But remember to do the NO SWEAT WARM-UP first!

## MAKING THE BED

Don't rush out of the house this morning without making the bed, as you are missing a great opportunity to tone up your legs!

This movement is based on a weight-training exercise called 'The Deadlift' and should be used whenever you make the bed or pick something off the floor, unplug the TV, dust the skirting boards etc. It is an excellent way to tone up the front of the thighs and bottom.

## 30. SHEET-TUCK TONER

For:  Toning the thighs and bottom
Coaching points:  Keep knees over toes
                  Do not go lower than 90 degrees
                  Make sure bottom stays higher than knees
                  Keep back flat
                  Look forwards and slightly down
Reps:  5–15

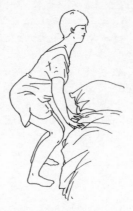

Stand in front of the bed, feet hip-width apart and toes pointing forwards or slightly turned out. Keeping your back flat and stomach pulled in, bend both legs so that you squat towards the ground. As you get lower down, hold on to the bed for support. Check that your knees stay over your toes and that you do not arch your back. Make sure your bottom stays higher than your knees, your shoulders higher than your bottom. Keep your heels on the ground. Never go lower than a 90–degree angle between your thighs and the floor. Look forwards and slightly down. Don't stay down in this position for too long or your legs will start to throb from a build-up of lactic acid. It is better to stand up and then squat down again several times if you can't tuck your sheet in in one go!

After you have tucked the sheet in, return to the standing position. Try to lead up with your shoulders. Make sure you don't hyperextend your knees as you stand up.

## 31. SHEET-TUCK TRICEPS TONER

For: Toning the backs of the arms
Coaching points:  Keep your head up and looking forwards
Keep your bottom close to the side of the bed
Keep your stomach pulled in, neck and spine long
Don't snap the elbows back as you straighten your
arms
Reps:  5–15

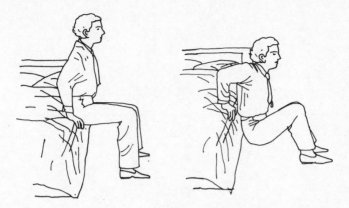

After you've tucked the sheets in, sit on the edge of the bed. Your knees should be bent with toes facing forwards. Lift your bottom so that you can place the palms of your hands shoulder-width apart on the edge of the bed with your knuckles facing forwards. Now lower your bottom towards the floor. Just before your bottom would touch the floor, raise your bottom up again until your arms are straightened but not hyperextended. Do not sit down on the floor or bed in between reps, but make sure you keep your bottom and back close to the side of the bed throughout the exercise. When you are strong enough to do 15 reps, make this exercise harder by sliding your feet further away from you.

## WASHING-UP

If your house is anything like mine, however much washing up you seem to do, it always seems that another pile of dirty dishes magically appears in the sink a little later! If this is the case, you should end up with a beautifully firm bottom and streamlined thighs!

## 32. DIRTY DISHES SQUAT

For: Toning the thighs and bottom
Coaching points: Don't go lower than 90 degrees
Make sure knees travel over the toes
Head up
Reps: 5–15

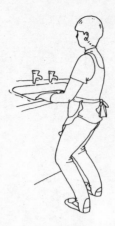

This is an excellent movement for toning up flabby thighs and bottoms. Do it when you are standing at the sink (washing-up, preparing vegetables etc.) as this will give you something stable and of an appropriate height to hold on to. But don't let the sink do the work for you! The push should come from your legs.

It does have such good results that I suggest you do it as often as possible – perhaps two or three times a day in the beginning. Once your legs get stronger you can do this squatting movement anywhere, just stretching your arms out in front of you for balance.

Stand feet hip-width apart, toes facing forwards or slightly turned out. Stretch your arms out in front of you to hold on to the sink for balance. Keep your spine straight, neck long and stomach pulled in. Bend your knees, carefully controlling your movement down, always checking that your knees travel over your toes. Keep your back flat and head up. As your legs get stronger you will be able to go lower. *Never* go lower than a 90 degree angle at the knee joint. Return smoothly to starting position, pushing up through the toes. Don't lock your knees back as you stand up.

Once you can do 15 reps easily, progress to the slightly harder exercise below.

## 33. DIRTY DISHES SQUAT LIFT

For: Toning the thighs and bottom
Coaching point: Tighten the buttock of the supporting leg
Reps: 5–15 each side

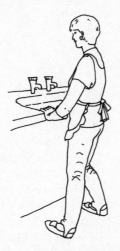

Stand, as in the Dirty Dishes Squat. This time, as you squat down push up again so that you transfer all your weight on to your right leg, while your left leg is lifted out to the side off the floor. Squeeze your right buttock as you do this. Make sure your left leg is straight with the foot flexed – you do not need to lift it more than a few inches off the floor. Keep your stomach pulled in and neck and spine long. Repeat on the other side for the desired number of reps.

## IRONING

As ironing is my pet hate out of the household chores, I've spent a lot of time inventing other exercises to reduce the tedium of it. If you have a big pile of ironing, try doing the following exercise in between batches – for example, five leg lifts after each batch of shirts! But please make sure you do turn the iron off while you're doing these.

## 34. IRONING LEG LIFTS

For: Toning the outer thighs

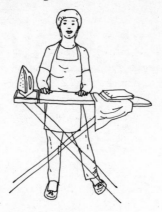

Coaching points:  Keep the supporting leg bent
                  Keep your hips pointing forwards
                  Stand tall
                  Don't arch your back
Reps:  5–15 on each leg, straight out to the side
       5–15 on each leg, slightly behind

Stand side on to the ironing-board, holding on to it with your inside
hand for balance. (Make sure the iron is turned off and out of harm's
way.) Pull up pelvic floor and tighten your stomach and buttock
muscles to give your lower body a firm support. Keep your spine
and neck long throughout. Bend the inside leg so it can provide a
solid base. Flex the foot of your outside leg and lift it out to the side
so that you can feel tension in the outside of your thigh. Keep your
hips square and facing forwards. Now lift and lower this leg a few
inches with a slow, controlled movement. Make sure you are only
using the leg and buttock muscles by keeping the centre of your
body (stomach, buttocks and pelvic floor) steady. It may help if you
place your outside hand gently on your stomach to remind you to
keep it tight and pulled in while you are doing the lift. You must not
arch your back. The actual lifting movement does not have to be
too big. Try to keep your leg long and stretched out as you lift. Stand

tall and don't lean into the ironing-board – it is there for balance, not support. Now swing your leg back a few inches and repeat the exercise in this new position so that you feel your buttocks work – keeping your stomach pulled in all the time. Repeat on the other side.

## WAITING FOR THE KETTLE TO BOIL

If the old adage 'A watched kettle never boils' is true, you should end up with a super-toned bottom. The following exercise is brilliant for firming up flabby bottoms.

### 35. THE BOILING KETTLE BOTTOM SHAPER

For: Firming the bottom
Coaching points: Knees bent
                        Don't arch back
Reps: 5–20 (until the kettle has boiled)

This movement can really be done anytime and anywhere although waiting for the kettle or toaster is ideal as it gives you a timer. Stand tall, spine lengthened and stomach pulled in, feet hip-width apart and toes facing forwards or slightly turned out. Don't lock your knees. Take a deep breath and exhale slowly, pulling your stomach in. Tighten your buttocks as hard as you can, pulling up on the pelvic floor. Don't arch your back. Hold for a couple of seconds. Relax. Repeat until kettle has boiled.

## SWEEPING THE FLOOR

How often do you sweep or mop your kitchen floor? If you want a trim, tiny waist, that floor should be kept spotlessly clean as every time you pick up a broom or mop you can do the exercise below.

### 36. SWEEPING AWAY THE WAIST

For: Trimming the waist
Coaching points: Keep hips facing forwards
Reps: 5–15 each side

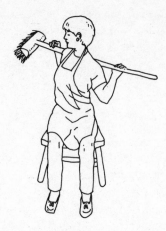

Sit on a kitchen stool or bench, feet flat on the floor directly below
your knees. Hold a long stick, mop or broom across your shoulders.
Pull up on the pelvic floor, tighten your stomach muscles and keep
your spine and neck long. Now gently swing from side to side so
that you stretch out the sides of your body. Keep your hips facing
forwards, let your head turn with your torso and keep your chest
wide and open.

## SCRUBBING THE FLOOR

OK. Now's the time to get down on your hands and knees and
scrub that floor! While you are down there, do the following bottom
throbbers. If you have young children you can also do this routine
while you are picking up their toys! If the floor is hard, put some
newspaper underneath your knees.

### 37. KITCHEN FLOOR LEGS AND BOTTOM ROUTINE

For: Toning the bottom and backs of the thighs
Coaching points: Keep your back flat and hips square
                          Keep the movements slow and controlled
Reps: 5–20 on each leg for all three parts of the routine

a. Kneel on all fours on the floor, pulling your stomach in and
keeping your neck and spine long. (You may find it more comfortable
if you put your hands together, bend your arms and rest your head

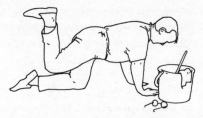

on your hands, but make sure that this does not cause you to arch your back.) Lift your right leg, so that the knee is bent and thigh parallel to the floor, with the foot flexed and facing the ceiling. Slowly and with control push your heel up towards the ceiling and lower it again for the desired number of reps. Do not raise your foot more than an inch or two. Concentrate on keeping the thigh parallel to the floor and hips square. Think of leading up to the ceiling with the sole of your foot and then pressing down to the floor, leading with your knee.

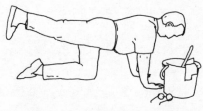

b. Now straighten your right leg out so that the whole leg is parallel to the floor. Slowly lift and lower the leg for the desired number of reps. Again, do not lift your leg more than an inch or two. Make sure this is a small controlled motion so that you don't arch your back.

c. Finally, curl your heel in towards your bottom and then press it out again so that the leg is as straight as possible and parallel to the floor. Repeat for the desired number of reps.

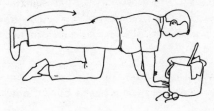

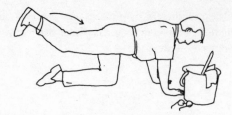

Now repeat this whole routine with the other leg.

## DUSTING

When was the last time you dusted those high shelves or that picture rail? Now's the chance to spring-clean your home while giving your body a lovely stretch up the sides. Remember – always warm up first!

### 38. DUSTER'S SIDE STRETCH

For:  Stretching out the side of your body and trimming the waist
Coaching points:  Keep knees slightly bent
Hold:  6–8 seconds on each side

Stand tall, stomach pulled in, spine and neck long. Stretch up to touch the door-frame or reach the cupboard by stretching right hand up above your head and feeling a stretch down this side of your body. Hold for 6–8 seconds. Keep your knees slightly bent. Repeat on each side.

## HOOVERING

One of the best times to stretch at home is after hoovering, as your muscles should be warm after all that moving about (remember to do the mobility movements before you start).

### 39. HOOVERING HIP STRETCH

For:  Stretching out the hip flexors
Coaching points:  Both knees at 90 degrees
                         Warm up first
Hold:  5–20 seconds each side

Switch off the hoover, hold on to it with both hands and kneel on the floor. Step forwards with your right foot so that it is flat on the ground with the knee directly over the ankle. Lean back slightly and tilt your pelvis forward so that you feel a mild stretch in the inside of your hips. Repeat on each side.

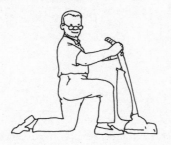

## 40. HOOVERING HAMSTRING STRETCH

For: Stretching out the hamstring muscles
Coaching points:  Warm up first
Keep hips facing forwards
Stick bottom out to feel more of a stretch
Hold: 5–20 seconds on each side

From the stretch position above, stretch your leading leg out in front of you so that it rests on its heel. Support your weight by placing your hands either side of your back leg on the floor. Stick your bottom out to feel a stretch down the back of the front leg. Repeat on each side.

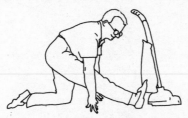

## 41. HOOVERING CALF STRETCH

For: Stretching out calf muscles
Coaching points:  Warm up first
Toes facing forward
Hips facing forward
Hold: 5–30 seconds on each side

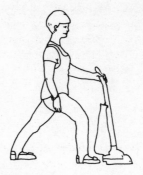

Stand feet together, stomach pulled in, spine and neck lengthened, holding on to the hoover with your left hand for balance. Now make a big step forwards with the right leg. Bend your right knee so that it is in line with your right toes. Stretch your left leg out behind you, pressing down through the heel so you feel a stretch in the calf muscle. Make sure the toes on both feet are pointing directly forwards and that your hips are square. Repeat on either side.

## 42. HOOVERING LOWER CALF STRETCH

For: Stretching the lower calf
Coaching points: As above
Hold: As above

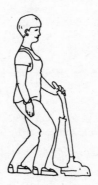

This area at the bottom of the calf muscle tends to be particularly tight and problematic in women who wear high heels a lot. Stand, holding on to the hoover for balance as above. Now step your left leg in so that your left toes are just a few inches behind your right heel. Make sure toes on both feet are pointing forwards and your hips are square. Bend both knees but pretend you put more weight on to your back foot so that you feel a stretch at the bottom of the calf muscle. Hold and repeat on each side.

## WAITING FOR THE TOAST!

Do something useful while waiting for your toast to cook in the morning. Most people have some spare wall space in their kitchen so use it to tone up your upper body while you wait.

### 43. TOAST AND TONE

For:  Toning the chest, shoulders and back of arms
Coaching points:  Hands level with shoulders
                  Back straight
Reps:  5–30

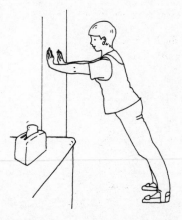

Stand facing the wall, about three feet away from it. Place your palms on the wall at shoulder height and shoulder-width apart. Slowly lower your body towards the wall, keeping your back straight and stomach pulled in. Don't arch your back. Then slowly push yourself out to the starting position again, being careful not to snap back the elbows.

Well done! You now know how doing the housework can be an ideal way to keep trim. Remember – all these exercises are flexible so you can change when and where you do them. For example, you could do the ironing exercise while you are washing up or vice versa, but you'll soon discover the best routine to fit into your lifestyle. Keep it up!

## THE SHOPPER'S SHAPE-UP

Carrying shopping is great exercise in itself, particularly if you walk round the supermarket with a basket and then carry it all the way home. Unpacking the groceries is also an excellent opportunity for toning up, as oranges, bags of flour, tins of baked beans and other cans are ideal to use for a little easy weight-training.

Start with just a few repetitions of each exercise, concentrating on good technique, and gradually build this up. As you get stronger you can also try increasing the weight (using heavier tins, bags of flour, etc.). If you've just walked home from the supermarket, you can go straight into the exercises below. Otherwise, do not forget to do the NO SWEAT WARM-UP in Part Three above.

### 44. SHOPPER'S TRICEPS TONER

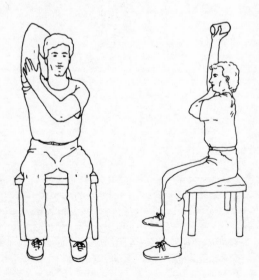

For: Toning and strengthening the back of the upper arms
Coaching points: Keep upper arm still
Elbow points towards ceiling
Don't hyperextend the arm
Keep back straight
Reps: 5–25 on each side

Sit on the edge of a kitchen chair or stool, with your stomach pulled in, spine and neck long, and feet flat on the floor, hip-width apart. Hold a tin or orange in your right hand and stretch up towards the ceiling. Keeping your elbow pointing straight upwards, drop your right hand behind your neck. Place your left hand just below your right elbow to check that the right upper arm stays still and right elbow stays pointing directly up. Now straighten your right arm, raising the hand so it points towards the ceiling again. Be careful not to snap the elbow back as you extend it. Concentrate on keeping your upper arm still and using your elbow as a pivot. Repeat for the desired number of reps. Change arms. Build up the number of reps gradually.

## 45. SHOPPER'S ARM CURL

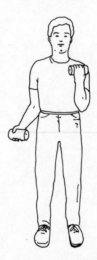

For: Toning and strengthening the front of the upper arm
Coaching points:  Keep upper arm still
                  Keep wrist straight
                  Don't hyperextend the arm
                  Keep back straight
Reps:  5–25 on each arm

Stand tall, knees bent, pelvis tilted forwards, stomach pulled in, feet
a little more than hip-width apart and pointing forwards or slightly
turned out. Hold a tin or orange in either hand, with your arms
straight down by your sides and palms facing away from you. Pull
your stomach in and keep your spine lengthened. Bend your left
elbow and curl the tin up to your shoulder, keeping the upper arm
still and close to the body and wrists straight. Slowly return the tin
to the starting position. Make sure you don't lock out the elbows on
the way down. Alternate the arms for the desired number of reps.
Build up the reps gradually.

## 46. SHOPPER'S ROW

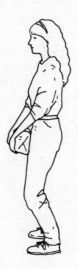 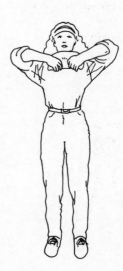

For:  Strengthening and toning the upper back, shoulders and front
        of the arms
Coaching points:  Keep the bag of flour close to body
                          Lead up with the elbow
                          Don't hyperextend arms on the way down
Reps: 5–25

Use a large object such as a bag of flour for this exercise. Stand with
your feet a little wider than hip-width apart, toes pointing forwards
or slightly turned out. Take the lock off the knees and tilt the pelvis
forwards. Pull your stomach in. Hold the bag of flour in both hands
with your arms stretched down in front of you. Your hands should
be two thumbs distance apart, knuckles pointing to the floor. Raise
the bag of flour to chin level, keeping it close to your body and
leading up with the elbows. Your elbows should end up higher than
the bag of flour. Lower the bag again slowly under control, making
sure you don't lock back the arms on the way down. Repeat for the
desired number of reps. Increase the reps gradually.

## 47. SHOPPER'S RAISE

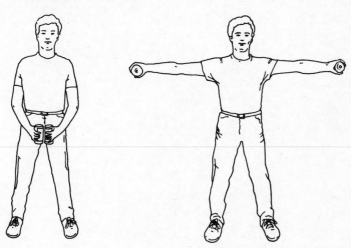

For: Strengthening and toning the shoulders
Coaching points:  Don't hyperextend the arms
                  Keep wrists straight
                  Try to keep the angle of the arms the same
                  throughout the exercise
Reps: 5–25

Stand with your feet a little wider than hip-width apart, toes pointing forwards or slightly turned out, holding a tin or orange in either hand. Pull your stomach in. Place your hands in front of your thighs, palms facing inwards. Raise both arms out to the side up to shoulder level or just above, keeping them straight and leading up with the knuckles. Keep the elbows slightly bent. Rotate the tins as you raise them so that at the top (i.e. shoulder-height) the tins are parallel to the floor and your palms are facing down. Return to the starting position slowly and with control. Repeat for the desired number of reps, increasing the number gradually over the weeks.

## 48. SHOPPER'S LUNGE

For: Toning and strengthening the front of the thighs and bottom
Coaching points:  Don't clench the tins or oranges too hard
                  Keep feet hip-width apart
                  Keep toes pointing forwards
                  Aim to achieve a 90-degree angle on both legs
                  Don't bang knee down on floor
                  Keep body upright

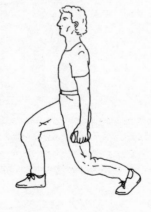

Reps: 5–25 on each leg

Stand feet hip-width apart, toes pointing forwards. Hold a tin or orange in either hand (NB: you may wish to do this exercise without the 'weights' for the first few weeks). Step forwards with right leg so that both legs can bend to 90 degrees. Don't bang the back knee on the floor. Keep your body upright and look forwards and slightly down. Your toes must stay pointing forwards. Keep your feet hip-width apart for balance. Relax your shoulders and arms – don't squeeze the oranges or tins too hard! Drive back with your right leg to the starting position. Keep spine and neck long, stomach pulled in. Alternate the legs for the desired number of reps.

## 49. SHOPPER'S LEG CURL

For:  Toning and strengthening the back of the thighs
Coaching points:  Keep hips pointing forwards
                  Don't arch back
                  Curl leg right up to bottom
                  Keep supporting leg slightly bent
Reps:  5–25 on each leg

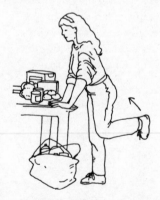

Stand tall, an arm's length away from the back of a chair, table or sink. Lean your upper body forwards slightly so that your back is flat and you can hold on for support. Bend your right leg slightly and curl your left foot up towards your bottom, your foot flexed.

The knee should stay pointing towards the floor. Slowly lower it again without touching the ground, resisting the movement as you do, and repeat for the desired number of reps on each leg.

## 50. SHOPPER'S SINGLE ARM ROW

For: Toning and strengthening the sides of the back and front of the arms

Coaching points:  Keep back flat and square
                  Support your body weight with your hands on your thigh
                  Keep wrist straight

Reps:  5–25 on each arm

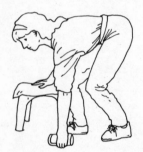 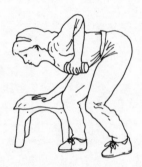

Place two tins on the ground in front of you and stand with your feet hip-width apart and toes pointing forwards. Bend your knees so that your hips lower towards the floor. Check that your knees stay over your toes and that you don't go down lower than 90 degrees. Check that your shoulders are higher than your bottom and your bottom is higher than your knees. Keep your back flat. Step about 1–2 feet forwards with your right foot (checking that your toes are still pointing forwards) and place your right hand on a stool or bench for support. Reach down with your left hand and draw the tin up to your armpit, leading with your elbow and keeping your arm close to your body. Lower it back down again slowly and with control – not touching the floor until the end of the reps. Make sure that you never hyperextend your arm on the way down and repeat on the other side.

## 51. ALTERNATE TIN PRESS

For: Toning and strengthening the shoulders
Coaching points:  Forearms stay vertical
                  Keep back straight
                  Keep knuckles up and elbows pointing down
Reps: 5–15

Sit on a chair, holding a tin in either hand. Slowly raise them to shoulder-level, with your hands about twice shoulder-width apart. Then, straighten alternate arms above your head so that the knuckles travel directly up towards the ceiling in a straight line. Don't lock the elbow out at the top. Your forearm should stay vertical throughout the movement and wrists stay straight. Lead with your elbow back to the shoulder-height starting position. Repeat, alternating arms for the desired number of reps.

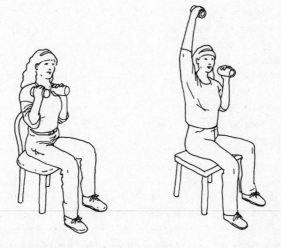

## 52. SHOPPER'S PEC DECK

For: Toning and strengthening the chest
Coaching points:  Don't arch the back
                  Don't hyperextend the elbows
Reps: 5–25

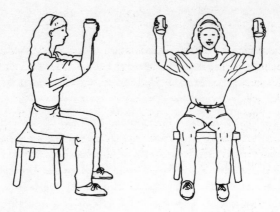

Sit on the edge of a kitchen chair or stool, feet flat on the floor, hip-width apart. Make sure that your stomach is pulled in and neck and spine are long. Holding a tin in each hand, press your elbows together in front of you so that your arms are touching, knuckles facing the ceiling and elbows pointing towards the floor. Keeping your arms at this angle, pull them apart, taking them out to your sides as far as you can without arching your back. Check that your knuckles always point upwards and your elbows down to the floor. Repeat for the desired number of reps.

Well done! You now see how shopping can keep you ship-shape. Remember the *No Sweat* principle of progression.

The man in the fable only became strong by lifting a bigger and bigger cow. Even if you just want to tone rather than build your muscles, gradually try to increase the number of reps you do. And keep shopping. You should soon have beautifully toned muscles!

# TELEVISION TONERS

If you're the sort of person who likes to come home and sit in front of the telly, don't worry. Below is the perfect TV work-out for you! So put away the popcorn and position yourself comfortably in front of the telly so you can tone up while watching your favourite programme. Watching television is a particularly good time to tone up flabby stomach muscles. Each movement will only take a few seconds, but remember – do the NO SWEAT WARM-UP – first or just dance around the living-room for a few minutes.

## 53. TV SQUEEZE

For: Toning the inner thighs and bottom
Coaching points: Keep back flat on floor
Reps: 5–25

Lie on your back, with your feet flat on the floor, hip-width apart and parallel and legs bent. Place a large cushion between your knees.

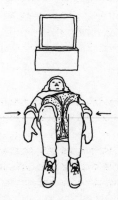

Breathe in. Breathe out, squeezing the cushion as hard as possible. Hold for a count of two and then slowly release. Repeat for the desired number of reps.

## 54. TV TUMMY TONER

For: Toning and strengthening the stomach
Coaching points: Keep lower back on floor
Reps: 5–25

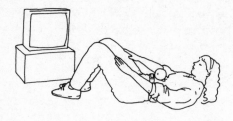

Lie on your back in front of the telly with your legs bent and feet
on the floor hip-width apart. Place an orange or grapefruit on your
tummy. Now slowly curl up, sliding your hands up your thighs and
looking at the orange as you do so. Don't lift your back off the floor,
and make sure the orange doesn't roll off. Don't worry if you can
only lift up a couple of inches to start with. As you get fitter you can
place your hands by your ears – but make sure you don't yank your
neck. Always return to your starting position with control. Don't just
crash back down – you want to work those tummy muscles both on
the way up *and* on the day down.

## 55. TV TUMMY TONER – WITH A TWIST

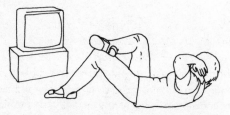

For: Toning and strengthening the sides of the stomach
Coaching points: Keep lower back on floor
                 Keep one elbow on floor at all times
                 Don't let the fruit roll off!
Reps: 5–25 on each side

Lie on your back so that the telly is to your right-hand side, legs bent, feet on floor hip-width apart. Place your right foot up on the lower part of left thigh (just below the knee). Put your hands behind your head and rise up towards your right knee with your left elbow so that you can watch the television programme! Keep your left elbow on the floor. Slowly lower with control and repeat for the desired number of reps before changing sides.

## TV CRUNCHERS

The following two exercises can be done with your lower legs resting on a settee or chair.

### 56. TV ABDOMINAL CRUNCH

For:  Toning the stomach muscles
Coaching points:  Don't yank your neck
                         Keep your hips directly underneath your knees
Reps:  5–25

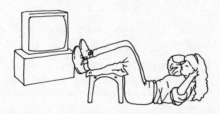

Lie on the floor with your lower legs resting on the settee or chair. Your hips should be directly underneath your knees. Place your finger-tips by your ears or loosely clasp them behind your neck and breathe in. Breathe out and slowly curl up, aiming to touch your knees with your elbows, and trying to flatten your stomach as you go. Breathe in and slowly curl down again, still trying to flatten your stomach. Do not rest on the floor in between reps – as soon as your shoulders touch the floor, curl up again.

## 57. TV ABDOMINAL CRUNCH AND TURN

For: Toning the sides of the stomach muscles
Coaching points: Don't yank your neck

Keep your hips directly underneath your knees
Reps: 5–25 on each side

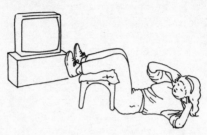

Repeat Exercise 56 above, but this time when you come up, touch your right knee with your right elbow and then reverse.

## 58. TV GUIDE PRESS-UP

For: Toning and strengthening the chest, shoulders and backs of the arms
Coaching points: Keep your weight over your hands

Keep fingers pointing forwards

Don't hyperextend arms on the way up
Reps: 5–30

Most people hate doing press-ups, but this is usually because they have poor technique. So, kneel on all fours and place your TV guide or something to read between your hands in front of you. You should be in a box position, with your thighs at right angles to the

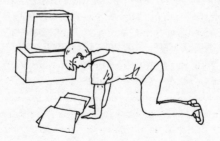

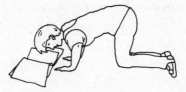

floor and your hands directly underneath your shoulders with your finger-tips pointing forwards. Keep your neck and spine long and stomach pulled in throughout the exercise. To the count of two, slowly lower yourself to the floor, keeping your weight over your hands so that you can read the words beneath you – indeed, your face should almost be touching them! Now slowly push upwards again to the count of two until your arms are straight but not hyperextended. Repeat for the desired number of reps.

## 59. TV THIGH TONER

For:  Toning and strengthening the outer thigh
Coaching points:  Don't arch back
                           Keep stomach pulled in
                           Isolate movement in the leg
Reps:  5–20 on each side

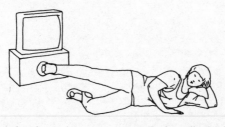

Lie on your left side so that you can watch the telly. Make sure you are in a perfectly straight line, bending the lower leg slightly to give a firm base. Support yourself on your left elbow (or lie down on your side with your left arm stretched out above your head along the floor). Pull your stomach in and flex your right foot. Stretch your right leg out as you lift it up towards the ceiling, making sure your upper body stays still. Lower the leg so that it is just above the supporting one and lift it again with control for the desired number of reps. This does not need to be a big movement – it just needs to

be isolated and controlled. Feel that you are lengthening your leg
every time you lift it. Repeat with other leg.

## 60. TV BOTTOM BLASTER

For: Toning and strengthening the bottom and outer thigh
Coaching points: As above
Reps: 5–20 lifts on each side
       3–10 circles clockwise
       3–10 circles anticlockwise

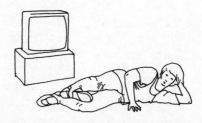

Lie on your side as in Exercise 59 above. Stretch your right leg out
and bring it forwards so that it is at as near 90 degrees to your body
as is comfortable. Flex the foot and lift and lower it with control for
the desired number of reps. Make sure your upper body stays still
and that your stomach and pelvic area are held firm. Don't let the
leg touch the floor on the way down, and always keep it lengthened.
Repeat for the desired number of reps. Now, keeping the leg swung
forwards, slowly circle it 3–10 times in a clockwise direction and
then 3–10 times in an anticlockwise direction. You will probably find
this difficult to start with, but build up the reps gradually, always
lengthening the leg through the heel before repeating the whole thing
on the other side.

## 61. TV BACK STRENGTHENER

For: Strengthening the lower back
Coaching points: Look down to floor
Reps: 5–15

Lie on your stomach facing the telly. Stretch your arms out with the
back of your hands resting on your buttocks. Slowly raise your head

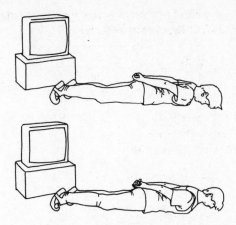

up, looking down to the floor at all times. Don't strain – this only
needs to be a few inches. Hold for a couple of seconds and then
lower slowly with control. Repeat for the desired number of reps.
As your back gets stronger you will be able to do this exercise with
your hands by your ears.

## 62. TV BOTTOM AND BACK STRETCH

For: Stretching out the bottom, outer thigh and spine
Coaching points:  Remember to warm up first
                  Hips stay pointing forwards
                  Keep back straight
Hold: 10–20 seconds on each side

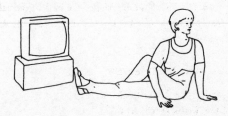

Sit on the floor facing the telly with your legs stretched out in front
of you. Place your left foot on the outside of your right leg. Sit tall,
with your spine and neck long. Turn to the left and push your right

arm against the outside of your left knee, turning the upper body round to the left so that you are looking over your left shoulder. Don't slouch. Hold for 10–20 seconds. Change sides.

## 63. TV GROIN STRETCH

For:  Stretching out the groin
Coaching points:  Remember to warm up first
                             Keep back flat
Hold:  10–30 seconds

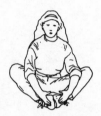

Sit in front of the telly with the soles of your feet flat together. Keep your spine and neck lengthened and pull up on your pelvic floor. Hold on to your toes and gently pull forwards, bending from your hips with a flat back. Gently push your knees down with your elbows, and hold for 10–30 seconds. As the feeling of stretch subsides, push down with your elbows a little harder.

## 64. TV STRADDLE STRETCH

For:  Stretching out the groin
Coaching points:  Don't round your back
                             Push yourself forwards on to your hips
Hold:  10–30 seconds

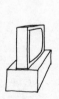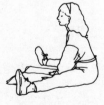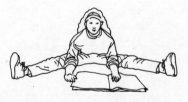

This is also a great exercise to do while reading the Sunday papers! Sit in front of the telly with your legs spread as wide as possible and the backs of your knees in contact with the ground. Keep your spine and neck lengthened. Slowly bend forwards from the hips. You may find it easier to put your hands in front of you for support. Don't try to touch the ground with your head – your spine and neck must stay lengthened. Instead, imagine that you are trying to touch the floor with your chest. Hold for 10–30 seconds and as the feeling of stretch subsides, lean forwards a little more. But don't worry if you can't lean forwards very much to begin with. The important part is that your back stays straight. Relax. Repeat.

Make a point of doing a couple of these exercises every time you switch the television on. You will soon tone up – rather than turning into a couch potato!

# THE BATHROOM WORK-OUT

Bathtime is supposed to be relaxing, but don't worry – the following exercises really are 'no sweat' and are a useful way to stretch out after a hard day.

I like to do these exercises after I have warmed up with a brisk walk and then taken a shower or quick bath. Although a hot bath or shower will warm you up, this will not warm the muscles thoroughly, so make sure you do some of the NO SWEAT WARM-UP exercises first. A quick jog around the house, up and down the stairs etc. should be enough.

## 65. LOO ROLL

For:  Releasing the spine and neck
Coaching points:  Support body weight by resting chest on thighs
Reps:  2–5

Sit on the toilet with your feet flat on the floor directly below your knees. Pull in the stomach, lift up the pelvic floor and lengthen the spine. Breathe in, stretching up to the ceiling with both arms. Breathe out again, slowly tucking your chin in and rolling down so that the spine is curved and arms slowly lower to hang loosely by your sides.

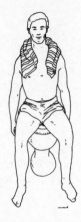 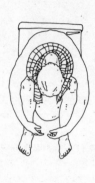

Don't just collapse into this relaxed position – control the downwards roll. Rest there a few seconds, supporting the body weight with your chest on your thighs. Breathe in again, rolling up slowly using the stomach muscles and feeling the spine stretch out again. Your head should be the last thing to come up.

## 66. BATHTIME PULL

For:  Stretching the hamstrings
Coaching points:  Your muscles will only be superficially warm from the bathwater so make sure you have thoroughly warmed up first
                Don't round your back
Hold: 5–20 seconds

Tight hamstrings are the cause of many back problems. Sit in the bath, legs stretched out in front of you and feet pressed up against the end. Pull your stomach in and keep your spine lengthened, stretching your arms out in front of you so that they are straight but still relaxed. Slowly stretch forwards imagining that someone is pulling your hands. Keep your spine straight, neck long and backs of knees pressed down. The chest and head should be lifted. Don't

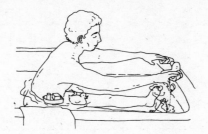

worry if you can't stretch forwards more than an inch or two to start with. Hold for 5–20 seconds, then slowly contract the stomach muscles to return to the starting position.

## 67. SINK STRETCH

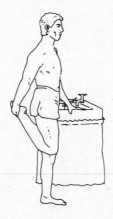

For: Stretching the front of the thighs
Coaching points: Again, make sure you are thoroughly warmed up
              first
              Keep supporting leg bent
              Check knee is pointing to the floor
Hold: 5–15 seconds on each leg

Stand tall, holding on to the sink with your right hand for support. Bend your left leg at the knee and pull your left foot with your right hand up towards your buttocks so that your knee is pointing straight down to the floor. You should feel a stretch in the front of the thigh – *not* in the knee area. Tilt your pelvis forwards slightly to increase the stretch, and keep your spine lengthened, lifting up from pelvic floor. Keep the supporting leg slightly bent to provide a stable base, and hold for 5–15 seconds on each side, repeating the stretch twice.

## 68. TOWELLING DOWN

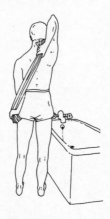

For: Stretching the backs of the arms
Coaching points: Always warm up thoroughly first
                 Don't arch your back
Hold: 5–15 seconds on each arm

Stand tall, spine and neck lengthened, holding a small towel above your head. Then drop your right hand so that the elbow is bent behind your neck. Your left arm should be straight down by your left side. 'Dry your back' by gently pulling with the left hand so that the towel is taut and you feel a stretch in the bent right arm. Hold for 5–15 seconds. Change sides.

Well done! You should have found plenty of exercises to do at home. Don't worry if you don't do them all at once. Try them as the right opportunity arises and always remember to keep concentrating on good technique, with your neck and spine long and stomach pulled in. You are better to do just a few exercises each day correctly than rush through a whole lot with poor technique.

# THE WORKER'S WORK-OUT

Work is one of the first things to interfere with a fitness regime. And you may not always be able to do something active during your lunch break or when you leave to go home. But don't despair! Even if your whole life seems to revolve around your work place, there are still plenty of opportunities to keep in trim – including the time spent getting there.

If you have a desk job it is particularly important to keep mobile because your joints will tend to get very stiff if kept in the same position for any length of time. The mobility movements in the NO SWEAT WARM-UP can easily be done in any work environment and will get the lubricating fluid in your joints flowing again, making you feel ever so much better.

This part is crammed full of exercises and tips to help make your working day all the more active. Remember – keep that neck and spine long at all times, with your stomach pulled in so that you improve your posture and tone your tummy at every opportunity.

## WORK TIPS

Before we look at specific exercises that you can do while commuting and in your work environment, below are some useful tips for combining exercise with a working life.

1. Get off your bus or train a stop early and walk the rest of the way so that you get your circulation moving first thing.

2. There is nothing like being late for work to make you move quicker! But even if you aren't late, always approach the stairs as if you are making up for lost time! Running up stairs and escalators is an excellent opportunity to tone your legs and is also an invigorating start to the working day. Remember – you may be sitting down for the next eight hours, so take this last opportunity to be really active. Think of yourself as a powerful

athlete and really go for it! However, never run up stairs or escalators if you are wearing high heels or carrying a heavy bag.

3. Instead of spending your lunch-hour in the pub, canteen or restaurant, go for a brisk walk in the park. Doing something active in the middle of the day will make you feel much more alert in the afternoon. Avoid doing anything too strenuous, though. You don't want to feel physically tired afterwards.

4. Take up an after-work sport with some of your colleagues. Badminton, tennis and squash are all sociable ways to keep fit.

5. Many offices realise how important it is for their staff to keep fit. If there is a gym at your office, use it to stretch out during your lunch-time.

6. Tell your colleagues that you are trying to get fit. This way they will not think you odd if you start doing some strange-looking movements at your desk. They may even be encouraged to join you!

7. Try not to sit still at your desk for too long at one time. Take a break at least every 90 minutes, preferably once an hour.

8. If you have to entertain a client, why not suggest something active? Some of the best business deals are done on the golf course. Alternatively, you could play squash, tennis or just have a swim and sauna.

9. If you are sitting at a desk all day, it is particularly important to follow the Posture Programme rigorously in this section. You will feel much less tense if you apply these posture principles throughout your working day.

10. Don't sit with your legs crossed as this restricts circulation and can aggravate varicose veins.

11. When talking on the telephone, never rest the receiver between your ear and shoulder. Always hold the receiver with one hand.

12. If you have to talk to a colleague, walk over and chat to him in person rather than phone him on the internal system. Similarly, when you send mail internally, use one of your breaks to deliver it by hand.

13. Try to use any time spent travelling to and from work to relax, concentrating on your posture and breathing.

14. *No Sweat Fitness* is not just about keeping active between the hours of nine and five! Try to incorporate some of the movements from other sections (e.g. THE HOME WORK-OUT) into your everyday life as well.

15. Remember – always follow the guidelines laid out in THE NO SWEAT WARM-UP before doing any exercise. Although you probably won't have the opportunity to do the whole thing in your work-place, at least make sure you mobilise the appropriate part of the body, or spend a few minutes walking around to raise your body temperature.

## THE COMMUTER'S WORK-OUT

Commuting, particularly in big cities, can be one of the most frustrating and futile parts of your day. With the *No Sweat Fitness* approach, however, it can be an invaluable opportunity to keep in trim. Try to be as active as possible in this period. If you only live a mile or two away from work, why not walk or even jog? In fact, I even have a friend who roller-skates through Regent's Park to work in central London! And if you don't see yourself as having *Starlight Express* potential, cycling is much easier, and, like skating, saves on transport costs while getting you fit. Your choice of transport obviously depends on changing/showering facilities at work, but many offices now provide showers so it may well, in fact, be feasible for you to jog or cycle there.

If you travel by bus, tube or train, get off one stop early and walk the rest of the way. Similarly, if you drive, park the car further away than usual and walk. A brisk walk before work really is an excellent way to wake yourself up and prepare for the day ahead. Alternatively, at the end of a hard day, walking home is a great method of unwinding and reassessing the day's events.

Below are some movements which can be done on your way to work.

## TRAVELLING BY CAR

If you drive to work you are in danger of arriving feeling tired and tense before the day has even started! To help minimise backache, make sure your car has a firm seat which supports the lower back properly, and possibly buy a lumbar support designed to be used in cars as well. Try not to grip the steering wheel too tightly or tense up your neck and shoulders. It is better for your spine if you sit close to the steering wheel with your knees bent rather than stretched out.

### PARKING TIP

If you do not have power steering, parking can be a prime opportunity to tone up those flabby arms. Make sure you use them to do all the work and avoid twisting the spine. Keep your feet flat on the floor, knees bent, stomach pulled in.

## TRAFFIC LIGHT TONERS

These exercises can be done anywhere – sitting on a bus, train or at your desk – because no one can see what you're doing. Indeed, with a bit of practice, you will even be able to do them walking along the street.

### 69. TRAFFIC LIGHT INTERNAL TONER

For: Strengthening the pelvic floor muscles
     Preventing stress incontinence
     Improving your sex life
Coaching points: Keep all your other muscles relaxed
                 Keep breathing
Hold: 5 seconds

Sitting at traffic lights is an excellent opportunity to do a little internal toning! Make sure you are sitting upright, with your neck and spine long. Now draw your muscles up inside, tightening them around your front, back and middle passages, imagining that there is a figure of eight of muscles inside. Try to keep all your other muscles relaxed and do not stop breathing. Hold for about five seconds. Repeat until the lights change.

This is an excellent exercise for women before and after having a baby and is also useful for men as it helps prevent that pot-belly look! Do it as often as you can!

## 70. TRAFFIC LIGHT BOTTOM FIRMER

For: Toning the bottom
      Strengthening the stomach muscles
      Improving posture
Coaching point: Do this as often as you can!
Reps: 5–15, or until the lights change

When the lights are red, check that you are sitting tall, stomach pulled in, spine and neck long, with your feet flat on the floor. Pull in your stomach muscles and clench your buttocks. Hold for a few seconds and release. Repeat until the lights change.

## DRIVER'S REFRESHER

When you park the car try doing some of the NO SWEAT WARM-UP mobility movements to wake you up and prepare you for the day ahead. Hip Circles (p54), Torso Twists (p56), Shoulder Rolls (p56), Arm Circles (p57), and Neck Rolls (p57) are all appropriate exercises to do when you step out of the car, and similarly you can do them at the end of the day when you arrive home.

## TRAVELLING BY BUS OR TRAIN

Commuting by bus or train can also be very stressful, particularly if there is some sort of delay. The following breathing exercise is an excellent way to calm yourself down if you are late! It can be done anywhere – in a bus, train or traffic-jam – and you should try to do it as often as you can so that it becomes part of your normal breathing pattern. For further breathing exercises also see pages 72–3.

## 71. LATE-TO-WORK BREATHING EXERCISE

For: Calming yourself down
　　Improving your breathing
　　Toning your tummy muscles
　　Improving body awareness
Coaching points: Concentrate!
　　　　　　　　Practise as often as possible
Reps: 5–10

Sit tall, feet flat on floor, spine and neck long. Slowly breathe in through your nose and let your stomach fill up with air like a big paper bag. Now breathe out, concentrating on pushing all the air out of your stomach so that the imaginary paper bag flattens and presses back against your spine.

### SHAPELY CALVES

The following exercise is a great way to develop shapely calves while standing on the escalator. If you are not doing this exercise, remember you should be walking or running up it instead!

## 72. CALF SHAPER (I)

For: Strengthening the calf muscles
Coaching points: Never attempt this if you are wearing high heels
　　　　　　　　or carrying a heavy bag
　　　　　　　　Keep your toes pointing forwards
　　　　　　　　Hold on to the side for support
Reps: 5–15 on each leg

Stand on the right-hand side of the escalator, holding on to the rail for balance. Place your heels over the edge of the step, making sure you are standing tall, with your spine and neck long, stomach pulled in and shoulders back. Rise up slowly on to your toes and then slowly go down again so that your heels drop beneath the step. Keep rising and lowering until you reach the top of the escalator.

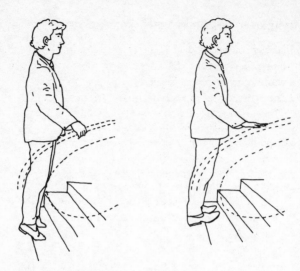

## 73. CALF SHAPER (II)

For: Strengthening the calf, shin and foot muscles
Coaching point: Sit tall
Reps: 5–15 on each foot

Sit tall, stomach pulled in, and neck and spine long. Stretch your left leg out in front of you so that the heel is on the floor with the toes flexed back. Now point that foot so that the toes touch the floor and the heel comes off. Continue pointing and flexing for the desired number of reps. Change legs.

## THE WORKER'S WORK-OUT

Whatever type of job you do, whether it involves sitting at a desk or standing at a counter, it is important that you do not stay stationary for too long at a time. Try to take an active break every 60–90 minutes, and the mobility movements in the NO SWEAT WARM-UP are an excellent way to limber up and stop your joints going stiff. Once you have warmed up, you can try the other movements below.

## 74. WORKING TRICEPS DIPS

An office chair is the perfect piece of equipment for doing these triceps dips. Make sure the chair is stable, though, and not going to wheel away. If you keep your lower body under your desk, your boss should not even be able to see what you are doing!

For: Toning up the backs of the arms
Coaching points: Keep the hands in line with the shoulders
Fingers point forwards
Avoid hyperextending the arms as you come up
Reps: 5–25

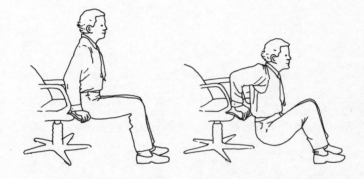

Sit on the edge of your chair and with your knees bent, feet flat on the floor, hip-width apart. Now hold on to the edge of the chair, with your hands close to your body. Slowly lower your bottom off the chair and dip down towards the floor. Go as low as you can without touching the floor, keeping your head up and stomach pulled in. Keep your bottom close to the chair so you brush up past it as you come up. Do not sit down in between reps. Keep going!

To make this exercise a bit harder, stretch your feet further out in front of you.

## 75. WORKING TRICEPS STRETCH

The Working Triceps Dips above are very strenuous so treat yourself to this good stretch afterwards.

For:  Stretching out the backs of the arms
Coaching points:  Don't pull on elbow joint
                              Don't arch back
Hold:  5–15 seconds on each arm

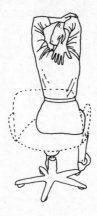

Sit tall, stomach pulled in and neck and spine long. Lift your right
arm straight up and reach for the ceiling. At the same time pull down
with your left arm towards the floor. Now use your left hand to clasp
your right arm elbow so that you can drop your right hand behind
your neck. Hold for 5–15 seconds. Do not arch your back – and pull
your stomach in. Release and repeat on the other side.

### KEYBOARD RELIEF

The stretches below are excellent for relieving office stoop. The first
one stretches out the trapezius muscle at the top of the back. The
second one balances this by stretching out the chest muscles which
often get tense from hunching forwards at a computer, word pro-
cessor or simply over the paperwork.

### 76.  KEYBOARD RELIEF (I)

For:  Stretching out the upper back
Coaching points:  Keep your chin tucked into your chest
Hold:  5–15 seconds

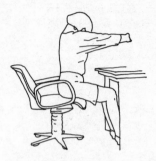

Sit tall, feet flat on floor, stomach pulled in. Stretch your arms out
in front of you, clasping your hands. Tuck your chin into your chest
so that you curve your upper back. Keep stretching through your
arms. Look down and hold for 5–15 seconds. Repeat if necessary.

## 77. KEYBOARD RELIEF (II)

For: Stretching out the chest
Coaching points: Keep stomach pulled in to avoid hyperextending
                 your back
Hold: 5–15 seconds

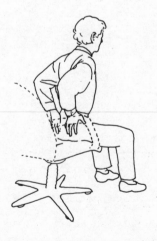

Sit tall on the edge of your seat, feet flat on floor and stomach pulled in, placing your palms on top of your buttocks. Press your elbows together, keeping your stomach pulled in and neck and spine long. Hold for 5–15 seconds and release.

## 78. TELEPHONE STRETCH

Talking on the telephone encourages you to hunch or tense up your shoulders – particularly if the business deal is not going well! When you put the phone down next time do some Shoulder Rolls (p56) and the following stretch.

For: Stretching out the shoulders
Coaching points: Keep arm at shoulder level
                            Avoid twisting your upper body
Hold: 5–15 seconds on each arm

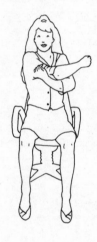

Sit tall, with your feet flat on the floor and stomach pulled in. Use your left arm to hug your right upper arm across the front of your body at shoulder-level. Don't twist your waist or torso and avoid pulling on the elbow joint itself. Hold for 5–15 seconds. Repeat on the other side.

## WRITER'S CRAMP

The following two exercises are my personal favourites for relieving writer's cramp, because if you do a lot of writing or keyboard work you will have a lot of tension in your wrists and forearms. As one of the exercises mobilises the wrists, you do not have to do a warm-up before starting. It is also very relaxing to give yourself a mini-massage in this area afterwards.

### 79. WRIST MOBILISER

For: Mobilising the wrists
Coaching points: Try to isolate the movement in the wrists
Reps: 5–10 clockwise
       5–10 anticlockwise

Sit upright in your chair, with your spine and neck long and stomach pulled in, resting your right elbow on the desk or supporting it with your left hand. Spread the fingers of your right hand and slowly circle it 5–10 times clockwise, then 5–10 times anticlockwise. Repeat this with the other hand.

### 80. WRIST STRETCH

For: Stretching out the wrists
Coaching points: Do the Wrist Mobility exercise above first
Hold: 5–15 seconds on each wrist

Sit upright as above, resting your right elbow on the desk. Gently push back the fingers of your right hand with your left hand. Hold for 5–15 seconds before repeating it on the other side.

### 81. DESK RELIEF

Sitting down all day puts a tremendous strain on your back, so try the following movement to keep your spine mobile.

For: Releasing tension in the back
Coaching point: Support body weight with chest on thighs
Reps: 2–3

Sit on the edge of your seat with your feet flat on the floor. Lift up and out of your hips and reach upwards towards the ceiling with

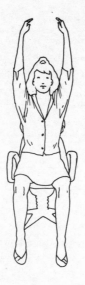
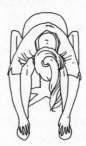

both hands. Breathe in. Now breathe out again, pulling your stomach in as you curl your chin towards your chest and down towards your thighs. Lower your arms and let them hang loosely by your sides. Keep sucking your stomach in every time you breathe out and rest with your chest on your thighs for a second or two. Return to sitting upright, keeping your chin tucked in so that your head is the last to come up. Repeat.

## 82. OFFICE EXTENSION

For: Shapely thighs
Coaching points:  Don't hyperextend the knees
                 Keep back straight and stomach pulled in
                 Hold on to sides of seat for balance if necessary
Reps:  5–20 on each leg

Sit on your chair with your spine and neck long, stomach pulled in and feet flat on the floor, hip-width apart. You may find it comfortable to lean back slightly into your chair so that your spine is supported.

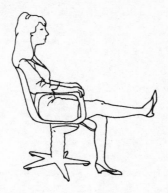

The back of your thighs should be pressed in to the edge of your chair. Keeping your upper body tall, slowly stretch out your left leg until it is as straight as possible, keeping your foot flexed all the time. Hold for a couple of seconds and then slowly press it down until your heel is *almost* touching the floor. Repeat lift and lower for the desired number of reps on the other side.

## 83. WORKER'S SIDE STRETCH

For:  Stretching out the sides of the body
Coaching points:  Don't lean forwards or back
                            Keep feet firmly on floor
                            Support your body weight on your thigh
Hold:  6–10 seconds on each side

Sit on the edge of the chair, stomach pulled in, back straight, feet flat on floor and toes pointing forwards, resting the palm of your left hand on the top of your left thigh. Reach up to the ceiling with your right hand, lifting out of your hips, so that you feel a gentle stretch down the right-hand side of your body. Make sure you do not lean backwards or forwards. Hold for 6–10 seconds. Relax and repeat on the other side.

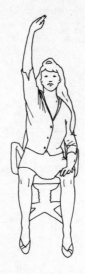

## 84. PAIN IN THE NECK

For: Releasing tension in the neck
Coaching points: Warm up with Shoulder Rolls (p56), Arm Circles
                (p57) and Neck Rolls (p57)
                Keep your shoulders down
Hold: 6–10 seconds on each side

Sit at your desk, spine lengthened and stomach pulled in. Keeping
your shoulders heavy and relaxed, slowly drop your head to the right.
Increase the stretch by gently pulling down with your left shoulder
at the same time. Hold for 6–10 seconds and release, returning
your head to the upright position, and checking that your neck is
lengthened (see Stand Tall p64). Repeat on the other side.

This exercise can also be done standing up, with your knees
slightly bent and feet hip-width apart.

## POSTURE PROBLEMS

Sitting at a desk all day puts a tremendous strain on your back. If you spend a lot of time hunched over a keyboard or papers it is easy to abandon everything you learnt about good posture earlier in this book. If you have bad posture, however, it can cause many problems, such as backache, a sore neck and shoulders, and digestive trouble, quite apart from making you feel dreadful at the end of the day. To release tension in your back, try the Desk Relief (p137), while the following exercise will help improve your posture as you work, as well as toning your bottom and stomach muscles.

## 85. OFFICE ATTITUDE

For:  Improving posture
      Toning the bottom and stomach muscles
Coaching points:  Sit tall
Reps:  5–10

Sit upright in your chair, with your feet parallel and flat on the floor. Keep your spine and neck lengthened and imagine that there is a piece of string attached to the ceiling and running down through your head, pulling your upper body up straight. Now squeeze your buttock muscles as tight as possible and pull in your stomach. Hold, and slowly breathe out. Keep squeezing your muscles and lengthening your neck and spine all the time. Relax and repeat 5–10 times.

## ON YOUR FEET

Standing up all day can also cause tension in the back and shoulders, often because you are standing lop-sided or arching your back. Keep practising the Standing Pelvic Tilt (p64) and the Stand Tall (p64) exercise for lengthening your neck. Even though you are not stooped over a desk, you may still be hunching your shoulders, so to relieve a tense upper back, try both Keyboard Relief exercises above (pp134–5) in a standing position with your feet hip-width apart and knees slightly bent.

If your job involves a lot of standing, you probably also suffer from throbbing feet at the end of the day. Standing still for long periods of time causes the blood to flow downwards, resulting in puffing ankles, tired feet and even varicose veins. Try to keep moving as much as possible, even if this just means transferring your weight from one leg to the other or walking on the spot. Relieve tension by doing the Ankle Circles (p52), Heel Raises (p52), Hip Circles (p54), Side Bends (p55) and Torso Twist (p56) that you learnt in the NO SWEAT WARM-UP. You may also find relief by doing the stretches (Calf, Lower Calf, Hamstring and Thigh) that you learnt in the WALKING PROGRAMME, but make sure you warm up first.


However you get to work and back and whatever your job, you now have the tools to relieve that build-up of tension and bring some activity into your work. You have no excuse now. So make use of this new freshness and energy when you get home in the evening – even if you do just give your dog an extra-long walk!

# THE FAMILY WORK-OUT

You have learnt how easy it is to incorporate more activity into your everyday life, both at home and at work. But if you have a family, you may feel you do not have enough time or energy to do all the other exercises in this book. Don't worry! This chapter is especially for you. Looking after children is actually an excellent opportunity to keep in trim. Children need to be encouraged from an early age to lead a healthy lifestyle, and this is where you can set a good example by following the guidelines and tips laid out in this chapter. Young children up to the age of ten will enjoy the specially devised WIZARD WARM-UP and ANIMAL CIRCUIT. Older children, on the other hand, will enjoy doing some of the other movements in this book with you, as well as going on family cycling trips, walks and rambles. Keep your children active and you will get fit in the process!

## CHILDREN AND FITNESS

We tend to assume that children are 'naturally' fit and healthy. Surely all that running around the playground at school and energy that parents find so exhausting must keep them fit? Unfortunately, this is not the case. Andy Jackson, who is a health and fitness expert, specialising in children's fitness, says that 'Children are actually some of the unfittest people in this country'. Many kids today are overfat and inactive. Add to this the fact that many of them smoke and have a poor diet and you paint a very gloomy picture for their future.

But surely all that PE at school should keep the children fit? Unfortunately, it is not as simple as that because often school PE is not the right sort of exercise for *health-related* fitness as it fails to meet its main components, as described in Part Two of this book – aerobic fitness, flexibility, muscular strength and endurance. Sports such as football, rugby, hockey and netball mainly develop what is called 'motor fitness', that is, the skill-related component of fitness – balance, co-ordination, speed, agility, power and reaction time. Although it is certainly beneficial to have good motor fitness, it is not essential from a health point of view. For health benefits, you need to think principally about developing aerobic fitness, as well as working on flexibility and muscular strength and endurance. School sports are not usually ideal for any of this. Although your child may be 'active', he or she may not be 'fit'.

Fitness in children is vitally important as it forms a good foundation for the rest of their lives. If you are obese (i.e. clinically overweight) as a child, then there is an 80 per cent chance that you will also be obese as an adult. However, as I explained in Part Two, aerobic exercise is an excellent way to prevent and control obesity, and while running up and down a hockey pitch will make you out of breath, it usually involves a lot of stopping and starting and is therefore not a good 'aerobic' exercise. Swimming, rowing, cycling and running are all more appropriate forms of exercise for conditioning your child's heart and lungs from an early age, while teenagers may prefer to dance or do special aerobics classes specifically designed for them.

Apart from controlling obesity and reducing the risk of coronary heart disease, aerobic fitness is important for children as it forms the base of the pyramid for later life. If you did not do any aerobic exercise as a child, you can only hope to see about a 15 per cent improvement in your aerobic fitness once you start doing aerobic training as an adult. If you were 'aerobically fit' as a child, however, you can see up to a 30 per cent improvement in later life, a similar pattern emerging when it comes to flexibility. If you want to improve your child's flexibility you should encourage them to do some gentle fun stretching exercises as often as possible between the age of five and ten (see ANIMAL STRETCHES below).

Strength training for children is a more complicated issue. Children under 16 should never do any form of heavy weight training as young bones are not fully hardened and heavy weights can cause malalignment in the joints. On the other hand, children still need to develop their muscular strength and endurance and can safely do exercises such as box press-ups that just involve their own body weight as a resistance.

It can be hard enough to motivate yourself to exercise, but with children you have to work extra hard, using your imagination and combining fitness work-outs with fun and games. If you tell your child to get down on the floor and do 20 box press-ups, they will probably either refuse point-blank and go off and play with their toys, or else get totally bored after just one or two. The trick is to keep their imaginations going. Instead of saying, 'Do a box press-up', why not say, 'Let's pretend to be an ant-eater. Get down on your hands and knees and dip your mouth down to the floor as if you were going to suck the ants out of the earth'? The more imaginative you can be, the more your children will enjoy it! You will be getting them fit without their even knowing it.

Encouraging children to get fit can be a lot of fun so why not join in and reap the benefits yourself? Below I have devised a warm-up routine for your children up to the age of ten, based on scenes from *The Wizard of Oz* and an aerobic and muscular strength and endurance circuit based on animal movements. There are, of course, many other ways to boost your child's fitness and the more you can join in the better. Older children will enjoy going on family cycling or rambling expeditions at weekends. Or why not book a family activity holiday this year – you'll be surprised how much fun this can be and the kids will be so occupied that it will be much more relaxing for you. And don't forget the local swimming pools and leisure centres. Most of them run special classes for children, from 'tumble tots' (fun and games for the under-fives) to swimming lessons.

Whatever you choose, I hope you and your children have a lot of fun!

# HOW ACTIVE AND HEALTHY IS YOUR CHILD?

Do the following questionnaire to find out how 'active' and 'healthy' your child's lifestyle is.

1. When your child comes home from school, how is he/she?

   A Very active – goes cycling, running around or straight out to play
   B Active – does not like to sit still for long
   C Semi-active – spends part of the evening doing something physically active and then sits down for a couple of hours to do homework/read/watch TV etc.
   D Inactive – sits down straight away to do homework/read/watch TV/eat and remains sedentary all evening

2. Does your child play any sport?

   A Yes
   B No

3. Does your child enjoy playing sport or doing organised games?

   A Yes
   B No

4. How many times a week does he/she play sport?

   A Three times or more
   B Twice
   C Once
   D Not on a regular basis
   E Never

5. Is this an aerobic sport (i.e. cycling, swimming, running, rollerskating etc)?

   A Yes
   B No

6. Do you have a dog?

    A Yes, and your child is involved in taking it for walks
    B Yes, but your child is not involved in taking it for walks
    C No, you don't have a dog

7. Does your child help you do the shopping?

    A Yes he/she goes with you to the supermarket and helps you carry the shopping
    B Yes he/she goes to the supermarket but does not help carry the shopping
    C No

8. If you take your family on an outing to a stately home, would you go for a walk in the gardens as well as look around the house?

    A Always
    B If the weather is good
    C Never

9. When you last went on a family holiday, would you describe it as 'physically active'?

    A Yes, very
    B Yes, we did do some physical activity
    C No

10. How would you describe your child?

    A Energetic
    B Average
    C Lazy or always tired

11. How would you describe your child?

    A Overweight
    B Plumpish
    C Average
    D Skinny

12. Do you know if your child smokes?

   A Yes, he/she smokes regularly
   B Yes, he/she smokes occasionally
   C No, he/she never smokes
   D Don't know

13. How often does your child eat chocolate, sweets, cakes, biscuits or crisps or drink fizzy drinks?

   A Very often – several times a day
   B Often – at least once a day
   C 4–6 times per week
   D 2–3 times per week
   E About once a week
   F Very rarely
   G Never

14. Is there a family history (i.e. in you or your partner or the child's grandparents) of any of the following – coronary heart disease, stroke, diabetes, cancer?

   A Yes – more than one of the above
   B Yes – one of the above
   C No

15. Does your child always eat breakfast?

   A Yes
   B Sometimes
   C Never
   D Don't know

16. How often does your child eat complex carbohydrates (e.g. wholemeal bread or pasta, potatoes, brown rice, vegetables)?

   A Every day
   B A few times a week
   C Rarely
   D Never

17. How often does your child eat 'fast food' (e.g. hamburgers, pizzas, milkshakes etc.)?

    A Every day
    B A few times a week
    C Rarely
    D Never

## ANSWERS

1. a = 5   b = 4   c = 3   d = 0
2. a = 2   b = 0
3. a = 2   b = 0
4. a = 5   b = 4   c = 2   d = 1   e = 0
5. a = 4   b = 0
6. a = 3   b = 0   c = 0
7. a = 4   b = 0   c = 0
8. a = 3   b = 2   c = 0
9. a = 3   b = 2   c = 0
10. a = 3   b = 2   c = 0
11. a = 0   b = 1   c = 3   d = 2
12. a = 3   b = 2   c = 0   d = -1
13. a = 2   b = 1   c = 0   d = 1   e = 2   f = 3   g = 4
14. a = 2   b = -1   c = 0
15. a = 3   b = 2   c = 0   d = 0
16. a = 3   b = 2   c = 1   d = 0
17. a = -2   b = -1   c = 1   d = 2

# RESULTS

## OVER 40 POINTS

Excellent! Your child is already leading a very fit and healthy lifestyle. He/she should thoroughly enjoy the NO SWEAT FITNESS routines in this section. Remember to join in with your child's activities. He/she should really be able to keep you in trim!

## 22–39 POINTS

Good! Your child is already leading a fairly fit and healthy lifestyle. This could be improved by following some of the FAMILY FITNESS tips below and by starting some of the routines in this section. Remember, this is all about family fitness, so join in as much as possible!

## UNDER 21 POINTS

At the moment your child is leading a fairly sedentary lifestyle. Following the guidelines of this part it should not be difficult to improve his/her lifestyle and start laying down the foundations for an active and healthy adult life. If many minus points were scored you must be careful that he/she is not running a high risk of coronary heart disease.

## FAMILY TIPS

1. At weekends do something 'active' as a family, whether it be cycling, a trip to the local swimming pool or leisure centre or a day out rambling in the woods.

2. Encourage your children to help with the more physical chores such as hoovering, washing the car or carrying the groceries home.

3. If you are worried about letting your child out to play or cycle alone, go with him/her! Or why not form a rota with other parents so you each take it in turns as to who supervises the physical activities.

4. Check your local paper for details of tumble tot classes and other activities that your child may enjoy.

5. Dance is an excellent form of physical and mental training for children. Don't forget that boys enjoy dancing too and there is certainly nothing 'sissy' about the hard physical training of ballet. Indeed, older children and teenagers may enjoy dancing or special aerobic classes.

6. Make your child's activity programme as varied as possible. Go swimming one week and play frisbee the next. Variety really is the way to keep your child interested in activity.

7. If your child is not naturally good at sport, explain to him/her that there are more important things than coming first in the school races. Many children are totally intimidated by sport at school and it can be very distressing if they can't keep up with their classmates, so take away the competitive element and encourage him/her to do some of the imaginative routines below. Let them see that fitness can be fun, or else they could be put off exercise for life. Only 3 per cent of the population continue doing sports from school in their 20s, and this figure drops to 1 per cent in their 30s.

8. Encourage your children to eat healthily from an early age. Kids love brightly coloured foods (hence the popularity of Smarties and coloured sweets) so if you are giving them a packed lunch, try to make the food look as inviting as possible, with colourful slices of tomato, carrots, red and green peppers, celery etc. Don't reward your child with unhealthy 'treats' such as chocolate, ice cream or sweets, as they are likely to associate such foods with 'comfort' eating later in life. Encourage older children to follow the NO SWEAT NUTRITION plan. Teenagers and especially girls, are often painfully self-conscious about their body shape and appearance in general, and need to be encouraged to eat healthily and stay trim for life rather than getting hooked on crash diets.

9. One in four smokers dies prematurely. And teenage girls tend to smoke more than boys – possibly because they think that it is a good way to control their weight while making them feel more sophisticated and grown up. The amount of cigarette advertising in women's magazines may also be a contributing factor. Explain to your children from an early age about the dangers of smoking and whatever you do, never smoke in front of them if you can avoid it. Encourage them to follow the NO SWEAT NUTRITION plan and explain how smoking will give them bad breath and skin.

Indeed, never smoke in front of babies or young children at all as this can cause chronic coughs and phlegm, with a high percentage of babies from households who smoke ending up in hospital during their first year because of bronchitis and pneumonia.

10. If you have a dog, make sure your child is involved in taking it for walks. Too many children are bought pets and are then never shown how to look after them.

11. If your child shows an interest in any of the movements in this book, encourage him to join in. And although the work-outs in this part have been especially devised for kids, older children may also enjoy the movements that you do to keep fit.

# THE WIZARD WARM-UP AND ANIMAL CIRCUIT

Below is a simple circuit of exercises designed to keep your child fit in a fun and entertaining way. If you tell your child the animal names of the movements and keep his/her imagination occupied, you should be quietly able to check that the movement is being done correctly.

## THE WIZARD WARM-UP

### 86.  LOST IN THE LAND OF OZ

Pretend you are Dorothy and walk around the room in all different directions, backwards and forwards and to the sides, as if you are lost. As you walk, shrug your shoulders up and down and pretend you are crying. Drop your head forwards and keep 'drying your eyes' with alternate hands.

### 87.  FOLLOW THE YELLOW BRICK ROAD

Pretend you are the Good Witch. Walking on the spot, turn your head to the right as if you are looking for the Yellow Brick Road.

Now turn your head to the left to look for the Yellow Brick Road. Turn your head to the right again and point in that direction with your right hand. Turn your head to the left and point that way with your left hand. Then point in front of you with both hands as if you have suddenly realised that this is where the Yellow Brick Road starts. Finally, whirl round three times to your left as the Witch did just before she disappeared!

## 88. SKIPPING DOWN THE YELLOW BRICK ROAD

Pretend you are Dorothy again. This time you have cheered up as you are on your way down the Yellow Brick Road to the Emerald City. Skip daintily in a big circle. Remember you are wearing the Wicked Witch's silver slippers so land gently on your feet! You don't want to damage those slippers! Make sure your heels lightly touch the ground.

## 89. THE SCARECROW

Now pretend you are the Scarecrow. Make all your limbs very floppy as you walk. Loosely shake your head, shoulders, arms, hands, legs and feet. Remember – you are very light as you are only made of straw!

## 90. THE TIN MAN

You are now the Tin Man! Move your limbs very carefully. You haven't been oiled recently so your joints are all rusted and you creak as you walk! Luckily, Dorothy has given you a tin of oil so pretend to lubricate all your major joints (your ankles, knees, hips, shoulders, elbows and neck). Now you can walk faster, lifing your knees high and marching your arms.

## 91. THE LION

Start growling and pretend you are the Cowardly Lion. Make big pouncing movements with your 'paws'. Prance around the room as if you are a big lion pretending to be very brave.

## 92. THE WINGED MONKEYS

Now leap around the room pretending you are one of the wicked winged monkeys who can fly. Swoop up and down as if you are attacking Dorothy and her friends.

## 93. THROWING A BUCKET OF WATER OVER THE WICKED WITCH

Pretend you are Dorothy defending herself and her friends. You have a big bucket of water that you keep throwing with a big sweeping motion over the Wicked Witch. Bend your knees as you throw the water.

## 94. THE WICKED WITCH IS DEAD — TOTO CELEBRATES

The Wicked Witch has dissolved on to the floor. Pretend you are Dorothy's dog Toto who is terribly happy that the Wicked Witch is dead. Run around the room like a dog, barking and waving a hand behind you as if you are wagging your tail!

## 95. DOROTHY RETURNS HOME

Finally, click your heels together three times like Dorothy to return home. Run around the room as if you were going across the fields back to Dorothy's house. Keep those knees high and swing those arms. Keep your back straight and head held high. Smile – remember you are very happy to be home!

## THE ANIMAL CIRCUIT

The following animal movements are designed to tone and stretch the body. They are meant to be done in a continuous circuit, so spend about 15–30 seconds on each movement. Children may particularly enjoy doing this in a group, so invite some of their friends round or join in yourself! Indeed, use the follow-my-leader approach, with the children copying exactly what you do, and these movements become an ideal opportunity for you to shape up at the same time. It is also more fun if you get your child to draw or cut out pictures of the various animals which can be placed as markers on the floor to remind them which animal they are going to play next.

I have included details of which part of the body each movement is working, although young children will probably be bored by this information so just keep their minds on the animals themselves. Making animal grunts, groans and noises will enhance the atmosphere!

For an 'aerobic' effect aim to do the circuit continuously for 15 minutes. So each exercise is followed by 'Riding the Pony', designed to keep the heart-rate up, which you can vary with dancing around the room, marching or jogging instead. Check that your child is working hard enough by seeing that he/she looks warm and is breathing fairly heavily. If your child looks exhausted or too red in the face, slow things down (e.g. walk instead of canter around the room).

Have fun, and remember to do the WIZARD WARM-UP first!

## 96. THE ELEPHANT

Aim: To keep the body mobilised and work the legs, bottom and shoulders
Suggested time: 15–30 seconds

March on the spot like an elephant with big heavy steps. Make sure your heels touch the floor. Now swing your right arm from side to side like a 'trunk'. Repeat with the left arm.

## 97. RIDING THE PONY

Aim: To keep the pulse rate high for an aerobic benefit
Suggested time: 15—30 seconds

Repeat this for 15 seconds after every exercise following. N.B. If your child looks tired, slow this down to a walk.

Canter around the room as if you were riding a pony. Remember to use your hands to control the pony's speed. Keep your back straight and make sure your heels touch the floor.

## 98. THE ANTEATER

Aim: To strengthen the muscles of the chest and backs of the upper arms
Suggested time: 15–20 seconds

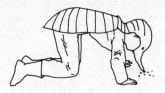

Kneel with your hands on the floor. Check that your hands are directly underneath your shoulders and that your fingers are pointing forwards. Keeping your back straight, lower your body so that your chin touches the floor like an anteater trying to suck the ants out of the earth. Press up to the starting position again, but make sure you don't lock out the arms when you straighten them. Keep the back straight at all times.

## 99. THE SEAGULL

Aim: To keep the pulse rate high and strengthen the shoulders
Suggested time: 15–30 seconds

Clench your fists and walk briskly around the room lowering and raising your arms at your sides like a flying seagull. Don't raise your arms higher than shoulder-height and keep the movements slow and controlled. Keep your back straight, and make sure your heels touch the ground.

## 100. THE DOG

Aim: To strengthen the muscles in the bottom and outer thighs
Suggested time: 15 seconds with each leg

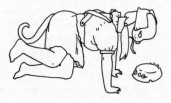

Kneel on all fours, hands underneath your shoulders, fingers pointing forwards. Keep your back flat and stomach pulled in. Now cock your right leg up to the side like a dog at a lamp-post! Make sure that this is a controlled movement and you don't arch your back. After 15 seconds change legs.

## 101. THE SHIRE HORSE

Aim: To strengthen the muscles in the bottom and front of the thighs
Suggested time: 15–30 seconds

Stand tall, feet shoulder-width apart. Raise alternate knees towards your chest like a shire horse who is trotting gracefully. Remember to stand tall and look straight ahead.

## 102. THE HONEY BEAR

Aim: To strengthen the muscles of the stomach
Suggested time: 15–30 seconds

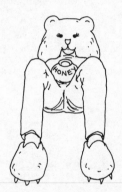

Lie on your back with your knees bent and feet flat on the floor. Imagine that you are a big cuddly bear with a giant pot of honey on your tummy! When you are lying down flat you can't see this honey so you want to curl your head up to find out where it is! Place your hands on your thighs and slowly curl up, letting your hands slide up towards your knees. Make sure your lower back stays on the floor and you keep looking upwards and forwards between your legs. Lower your back down to the starting position again under control.

## 103. THE KANGAROO

Aim:  To strengthen the muscles in the legs and bottom and develop
       explosive power
Suggested time: 15–30 seconds

Spring around the room like a kangaroo. Make sure you land lightly
with your heels down – remember you have a baby kangaroo in your
pouch! Keep your head up and looking forwards.

## 104. THE GORILLA

Aim:  To strengthen the muscles of the upper thighs, bottom and
       front of the arms
Suggested time: 15–30 seconds

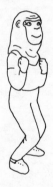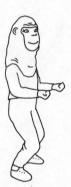

N.B. If your child looks tired, slow this down to a walk. Stand with
your feet hip-width apart like a big strong gorilla. Lower your bottom
towards the floor. Check that your knees stay over your toes and
that your thighs do not go lower than 90 degrees to the floor. Squat
slowly up and down. At the same time curl your arms up as if you
were banging your chest with your fists. Try to keep your elbows in
by your sides and hit the outside of your chest near your armpits.

### COOLING THE PONIES DOWN

After this ANIMAL CIRCUIT, it is now time to cool down. Canter
your pony round the room for about 30 seconds. Then slow this

down to an easy trot (for 30 seconds) and then down to a walk (for 30 seconds). If your child still looks red and breathless, keep him/her walking round the room for longer.

## THE ANIMAL STRETCHES

Now is a good time to do some simple ANIMAL STRETCHES. If the room you are exercising in is not very warm, make sure your child puts another layer of clothing on as the body will be cooling down quite quickly.

Don't start the stretches until your child has calmed down. Encourage the child to 'sneak' slowly and quietly into the animal positions (i.e. stretches), telling them that if they move jerkily or go into position too quickly they will 'scare the animals off'.

## 105. THE STORK

Aim:  To stretch out the front of the thighs
Suggested time: 10–15 seconds on each leg

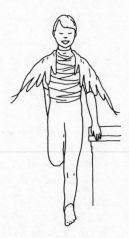

Holding on to a wall, table or friend for balance, stand on one leg like a stork, foot flat on the floor. Bend your other leg so that you can hold it by the ankle and pull it up to your bottom. Make sure the knee is pointing towards the floor. Stand tall. Hold for 10–15 seconds. Change legs.

## 106. THE CHEETAH

Aim: To stretch out the calf muscles
Suggested time: 10–15 seconds on each leg

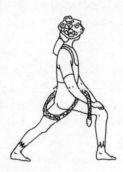

Stand with your feet hip-width apart. Step forwards with the right leg so that your right knee is bent and your left leg is stretched out straight behind you like a cheetah ready to pounce. Make sure the toes of both feet are pointing forwards. You should feel a mild stretch down the back of your left leg. Hold for 10–15 seconds. Change legs. Stay in this position and move straight into the 'Giraffe'.

## 107. THE GIRAFFE

Aim: To stretch out the backs of the upper legs – the hamstrings
Suggested time: 10–15 seconds on each leg

Stay in the Cheetah above. Now bend your back leg and straighten your front leg with your foot flat. Place both hands on the thigh of your bent leg for support. Now lean your body forwards so that you feel a stretch down the back of the front leg. Hold for 10–15 seconds. Change legs.

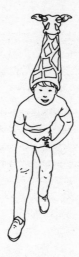

## 108. THE PELICAN

Aim: To stretch out the muscles of the upper back
Suggested time: 10–15 seconds

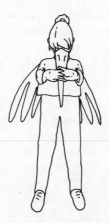

Stand, feet hip-width apart, knees slightly bent. Clasp your hands and stretch your arms out in front of you like a pelican's long beak. Drop your chin towards your chest and feel a stretch down the back of the neck and upper back.

## 109. THE MONKEY

Aim: To stretch out the backs of the upper arms
Suggested time: 10–15 seconds on each arm

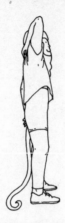

Stand like The Pelican above but with your arms hanging loosely by your sides. Now raise your right arm towards the ceiling. Keeping your elbow pointing upwards, drop your hand down behind you as if you were a monkey trying to scratch your back! Hold for 10–15 seconds. Change arms.

## 110. THE CHIMP

Aim: To stretch out the groin
Suggested time: 10–15 seconds

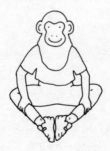

Sit on the floor like a chimp, with the soles of your feet touching
and pulled in towards your groin. Sit up tall, with your back straight.
Lean forwards to feel a stretch in the groin. Hold for 10–15 seconds.

## 111. THE COBRA

Aim:  To stretch out the stomach
Suggested time: 10–15 seconds

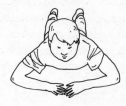

Lie on the floor on your stomach. Place your palms on the floor just
under your chin so that they form a triangular shape. Keeping your
elbows on the floor, push up on your arms so that your chest comes
off the floor and you look like a cobra. Look straight ahead. Slowly
lower.

## 112. THE CAT

Aim:  To stretch out the stomach and back
Suggested time: 10 seconds in both positions

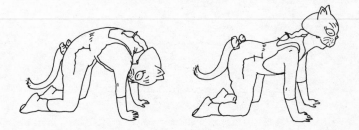

Kneel on all fours, with your hands directly underneath your shoulders and your fingers pointing forwards. Now pull up your stomach

muscles, drop your head and arch your back up like a cat stretching. Hold for 10 seconds. Now slowly lower your stomach and chest towards the floor so your back is arched, your head raised and neck lengthened. Avoid tilting your head backwards. Hold for a further 10 seconds.

## 113. THE STARFISH

Aim: To stretch out the whole body
Suggested time: 10 seconds

Lie on your back with your arms and legs apart in a starfish position. Stretch out both your arms and your legs. Hold for 10 seconds. Relax.

## THE ANIMALS WAKE UP

Finally, you need to wake your child up or else he/she may feel very drowsy and unco-ordinated after all that slow stretching. The best way to do this is to get them to pretend to be their favourite animal and just walk around the room or house stretching and moving their limbs as if they had just woken up. Alternatively, if there are several children doing the work-out you could have them form a 'crocodile' and walk around the house.

You don't want to get them too excited again so keep this part of the work-out to a minimum (i.e. not more than one minute). As you can see, children's work-outs can be fun. Try to encourage them to think of exercise as a game and soon they should be fit for life.

# NO SWEAT SPORT

*No Sweat Fitness* is all about being 'active' with minimal effort. It is about incorporating more physical action into your everyday lifestyle. Taking up a sport is certainly an excellent way to increase your activity level, but it must be something you enjoy. If anything is a chore you will never make it part of your life, so it's no good playing a sport just because you know it's good for you. If you don't enjoy it, you will never stick to it.

Allow yourself to be a 'sporting butterfly' for a while. There are so many activities to choose from that even if you consider yourself totally 'unsporty' you are bound to find at least one that you like and that fits in with your lifestyle.

It doesn't matter what you choose – every type of activity (done properly) has its benefit. So, if you've always dreamt of fencing like Errol Flynn or if Bruce Lee was your childhood idol, now is the time to start. Similarly, if you've always wanted to perform in *Starlight Express*, why not learn to rollerskate? Or what about learning to stomp your feet and click your castanets in a flamenco dance class or improving your sex-life with belly dancing?

However, make sure whatever activity you decide to pursue, it is something that you can afford to keep up and that is easily accessible. Don't make the mistake of getting hooked, for example, on watersports if you don't have a car and live miles from any inland water or the sea.

Below is an alphabetical list of activities, selected for the variety of fitness benefits they represent.


## AQUA FITNESS

GOOD FOR: FLEXIBILITY
AEROBIC CONDITIONING
PREGNANT WOMEN

Aqua fitness or water aerobics is a fun way of working out in water either at a class or on your own in a swimming pool or in the sea. The water both supports the body (so reducing the chances of injury) and provides resistance to work against, and it is a particularly pleasurable way to get fit as you feel so free and mobile in the water – probably the closest you will get to the sensation of walking in space.

You only weigh one tenth of your body weight in water, so it is ideal for pregnant women or anyone who is very overweight. However, aqua fitness is still hard work as water is a thousand times denser than air and provides a lot of resistance, a resistance which increases as you increase your work-rate.

Water has what is called a 'double positive' effect, which means that it works opposing sets of muscles. In other words, one simple movement can tone both the back and front of the leg.

Nevertheless, your heart actually drops 12–17 beats per minute as soon as you enter the water, so you will have to work that bit harder to get an aerobic effect. Try to incorporate lots of large sweeping arm movements as this will put your heart rate up, and you can also try fast walking (forwards, backwards and sideways), skipping and jumping through the water. Remember – for an aerobic benefit you need to keep moving quite vigorously for about 15 minutes. So, to increase the resistance of the water, just move faster or wear a pair of flippers. One way of toning the arms and chest is to keep pushing a beach ball up and down under the water, and you can even buy special hand paddles from big sports shops nowadays.

The good thing is, that you don't have to be able to swim to do aqua fitness as there is no need to go any deeper than chest-level. Make sure, however, that the part of your body that you want to exercise is always submerged, and always make sure you warm up first with 5–10 minutes' walking or jogging or by swimming across the pool.

## CYCLING

GOOD FOR:  AEROBIC CONDITIONING
           STRENGTHENING THE CALVES AND BACKS OF THE
             UPPER LEGS
           GETTING RID OF BODY FAT

If you enjoy cycling you are lucky as it is a sport that not only keeps you in shape, but also doubles up as a form of transport: in big cities it is often the quickest way of getting from A to B! It is also a good form of aerobic conditioning and does wonders for toning up the backs of the thighs, calves and bottom. You are unlikely to build up bulky muscles unless you start cycling competitively and have to tackle more speed work and hills.

For fitness benefits you need to pedal at a frequency of about 70 crank revolutions per minute. Try not to cycle in too high a gear. Pregnant women may not want to risk the open road but can still enjoy the fitness benefits of this sport on a stationary bike. The supported, non-impact characteristics of cycling are perfect when you are pregnant.

The main hazards of cycling are cars and other cyclists on the road, so make yourself visible with bright clothing and reflective bibs and be observant of what is happening all around you. Indeed, unattractive though they are, a few pounds invested in a cycle helmet might just save your life. Most injuries to cyclists happen within 20 yards of an intersection so be particularly careful at crossroads and junctions.

When buying a bike go to a specialist shop for advice and buy the best you can afford. It really is important for safety and comfort that the bike is suitable for you. If you are only going to cycle short distances, a 'sit up and beg' bike is adequate. If you suffer from back problems you may find the hunched-up position adopted on a racing bike aggravating, and while mountain bikes are expensive, they are delightful to ride both on and off the beaten track.

## DANCE

GOOD FOR:  FLEXIBILITY
           STRENGTH
           STAMINA
           CO-ORDINATION
           BALANCE
           POSTURE
           AEROBIC CONDITIONING

Dancing is one of the most natural and enjoyable ways to keep fit, and most types give you all-round physical conditioning as well as mental discipline. There is also tremendous scope on offer as there are so many different styles, such as ballet, jazz, ballroom, tap or even just bopping around the living-room.

One of the best types from a health point of view is belly dancing, or *raks sharki* as it is known in Egypt. Full of Eastern Promise, it is perfect for the well-endowed – the more you've got to shake and shimmy, the better! One teacher told me that her favourite build for belly dancing is a generous size 16 ('large ladies have the edge'), but whatever your size or shape, it will firm and tone all parts of the body, particularly the thighs, bottom, waist, hips, breasts and abdominal muscles. The gentle shimmying movements are good for your circulation and skin tone while the pelvic tilts and abdominal rolls can help relieve period pains and premenstrual tension. The ancient Egyptians even claim that *raks sharki* massages the internal organs and so can help everything from constipation to incontinence.

In the West, belly dancing still has the rather sleazy image of cheap titillation and raunchy cabaret, but it actually originated in the harem where it was performed *for* women *by* women, and in certain parts of the Middle East, it is still used as a 'birth dance'. The squatting woman in labour is surrounded by a circle of female friends who belly dance in order to encourage and stimulate her into giving birth. And even in this country belly dancing is sometimes taught as a pre- and post-natal exercise.

## FENCING

GOOD FOR:  POSTURE
BALANCE
CO-ORDINATION
REACTION TIMES
MENTAL DISCIPLINE
AGILITY
SELF-CONFIDENCE
STRENGTH (PARTICULARLY IN THE FRONT OF THE
THIGHS AND BOTTOM)

Fencing is often compared to chess as it is such a mentally stimulating sport. You need total concentration to master the complicated foot-work and plan a strategy of attack and counter-attack, and it is one of the more demanding sports to learn as you need to practise two or three times per week. Indeed, it may take you a year before you really get a feel for it, and in some of the stricter fencing academies in Europe, students are not allowed to pick up a foil until they have spent this length of time just learning the footwork.

## GOLF

GOOD FOR:   TONING THE LEGS AND BOTTOM (ALL THAT WALKING!)
            RELAXATION
            HAND TO EYE CO-ORDINATION

The main benefit of golf is that it gets you out into the fresh air and involves a lot of walking. It is also a very sociable way to do business and a good way to relieve executive stress. If you play a lot of golf, be careful that you don't overdevelop one side of the body. Counteract this by doing strengthening exercises for the side you don't use. You also need to do some stretching for the shoulders, arms and back.

## HORSE RIDING

GOOD FOR:   STRENGTHENING THE LEG MUSCLES, PARTICULARLY
               THE INNER THIGHS
            POSTURE (STRENGTHENS THE STOMACH AND BACK
               MUSCLES)
            BALANCE AND CO-ORDINATION

Horse riding is one of the most invigorating and enjoyable activities that can be done by people of all ages, shapes and physical abilities. It is one of those sports where you really do need good tuition from the start, both to be fair to yourself and the horse! From a fitness point of view, horse riding will improve your posture, and strengthen your legs, back and stomach muscles. It does not really have any aerobic benefit (the poor horse does most of the cardiovascular work!) unless you are of a very good standard and competing cross-country.

## JOGGING

GOOD FOR:  AEROBIC CONDITIONING
           BURNING FAT
           TONING THE LOWER BODY

If you enjoyed THE WALKING PROGRAMME in Part Two, the natural progression is to try jogging. This is one of the cheapest and most natural ways to keep fit and will ensure that you get masses of fresh air, a healthy complexion through better circulation and beautifully toned legs. People who are not used to running often say that they don't do it because it is so boring. If you run at a comfortable pace it is actually incredibly relaxing as it enables you to switch on to a mental autopilot and use it as a form of meditation.

Jogging is also an ideal way to No Sweat Fitness as it is so easily adapted into everyday life. Once you have invested in a good pair of running shoes (women will also be more comfortable wearing a special sports bra), you can run totally free of charge, whenever and wherever you want. It's ideal for people who do a lot of travelling as you can do it wherever you happen to be and it is a great way to get your bearings in a new town or location.

In order to avoid injuries, a good pair of running shoes is essential, and you should always warm up properly first, doing the stretches from THE WALKING PROGRAMME. It is equally important to spend five minutes or so cooling down and stretching out again afterwards because if you stop any aerobic exercise suddenly, you may well be endangering your heart. Good technique when you actually jog will also help prevent injury. Check that your stomach is pulled in, your neck and spine are long and your hips square, making sure you don't rotate your knees inwards or outwards as you go and that you always land with your whole foot on the ground – not just the toes.

The best way to start is to go out for about half an hour and alternate brisk walking (at about 15 minutes per mile) with slow jogging (at about ten minutes per mile) – any faster than nine minutes a mile is considered running. The most common mistake that people make is to roar off at lightning speed to begin with, only to be worn out a couple of minutes later. You will burn up more calories running at a low intensity for a longer period, so if you can't maintain a comfortable conversation while you jog, you are running too fast.

As you get fitter you can gradually increase the proportion of time you spend jogging. However, don't increase the mileage by more than about ten per cent a week, for although you can get aerobically fit quite quickly, the muscles and joints take longer to adapt to the new work-load. And for fitness benefits, there is really no need to jog more that about 12 miles a week.

If you live in a city, the best time to run is early in the morning, before the pollution has had a chance to settle. Running on grass will reduce the impact of your foot on the ground and running in woodlands and green areas will reduce the amount of carbon dioxide that you inhale.

And of course, if you don't enjoy running on your own, you could always try joining a local running group.

## MARTIAL ARTS AND JUDO

GOOD FOR:  STRENGTH
FLEXIBILITY
POSTURE
SELF-CONFIDENCE
SELF-DEFENCE

If you take up a martial art you have the double benefit of getting fit while learning how to defend yourself. All martial arts are steeped in tradition, many with religious and spiritual sides to them. Unlike some sports, taking up a martial art is a major commitment and it may take a year or more before you feel you are getting anywhere. The training can be very draining as you have to practise a movement again and again until it becomes spontaneous – so this is not the sort of activity for anyone with a low boredom-threshold. You must also be careful that you don't suddenly think you are Superman. False confidence in a real-life situation can be just as dangerous as having no confidence at all.

Judo is not strictly speaking a martial art, although it is still an excellent form of self-defence, more concerned with grabbing and throwing than striking. One of the most important things is learning how to fall properly, so expect to get lots of bruises!

## RACQUET SPORTS

GOOD FOR: HAND–EYE CO-ORDINATION
SPEED
STRENGTH IN THE ARMS AND SHOULDERS
AGILITY

If you're competitive by nature, you will probably find racquet sports an ideal way to keep active. The first thing you need to do is find a partner of the same (or marginally better) standard and most local clubs and sports centres keep names and addresses of people looking for partners. The main expense in racquet sports is always club membership, but most local authorities do have cheap public facilities.

Racquet sports are weight-bearing exercises so they reduce the risk of osteoporosis (brittle bone disease) by helping to increase bone density. However, avoid overdeveloping yourself on the racquet side of the body by doing some more intensive training (such as with weights) on the other side to balance this. Squash is the most demanding of the racquet sports and is not suitable if you are unfit or suffer from high blood pressure or heart problems. The 'stop start' nature of these sports means that they are not aerobically beneficial in the fullest sense.

## ROWING

GOOD FOR: AEROBIC CONDITIONING
STRENGTHENING THE BACK, THIGHS AND ARMS
FLEXIBILITY OF THE BACK

Rowing is one of the best sports for all-round fitness. It will condition your heart and lungs, tone up your whole body and burn up lots of fat. At competitive level, men can eat 5,000 calories or more without putting on weight and women up to 4,500. It is also a low-impact sport (your body weight is supported) so injuries are minimal.

Rowing is a good choice if you don't like solitary sports as it encourages a great sense of camaraderie and team spirit. You will need to join a local club – most of them will let you try a few sessions before committing yourself – and there are also special clubs for women.

## SWIMMING

GOOD FOR: Aerobic conditioning
Muscular strength and endurance
(particularly in the upper body)
Flexibility
Relaxation
People with breathing problems

Swimming is one of the most relaxing and natural ways to exercise and from a health point of view it is a very safe and unstressful way to strengthen your heart and lungs. To achieve this aerobic effect, however, you do need to be a good enough swimmer to swim continuously for 15 minutes or more, so it may be worth investing in a few lessons at your local pool to improve your technique. Many people don't know how to breath efficiently in the water so they get tired out very quickly – a good instructor should correct this.

As swimming is a non-weight bearing exercise, it is ideal for pregnant women, the disabled, elderly people or anyone with an injury. It is also a very comfortable way for overweight people to exercise (you are only a tenth of your body weight in the water). Unfortunately, swimming is not an ideal way to lose body fat as the very nature of the activity encourages you to store it to help make you more buoyant! If you are overweight, I suggest you go swimming for the aerobic benefits but also follow the nutrition guidelines later in the book (NO SWEAT NUTRITION) and do some other aerobic activity such as walking (see pp74–5) in order to lose body fat.

As with any exercise, remember to warm up and mobilise the body before you start. You should be able to do many of the mobility exercises in this book in the water. Try to vary your strokes as much as possible (alternating between breast-stroke, crawl and back-stroke) as this incorporates more muscles, so increasing the fitness benefits and minimising the chance of injury. Also, remember to cool down properly again afterwards. Overuse of the shoulder region can lead to tendonitis (inflammation of the tendons), so pay particular attention to stretching out the upper body at the end of your swim. Again, there is no reason why you cannot do your stretches in the pool or sitting on the edge.

## TEAM SPORTS

GOOD FOR:  CO-ORDINATION
CAMARADERIE
HAND—EYE CO-ORDINATION
AGILITY
SPEED

There are so many team sports, including football, hockey, lacrosse, netball, volleyball and rugby, that you could write another book on their fitness benefits. For many people, this sort of sport is the most enjoyable way to keep fit as it is so sociable. Most of the ones that involve charging up and down a muddy pitch (such as football, rugby and hockey) are good for stamina building although as they usually involve a fair amount of stopping and starting (depending on the skill of the team!) they are not so good for aerobic training. The area of body strengthened obviously depends on which sport you choose (i.e. football tones up the legs, whilst volleyball strengthens the arms, shoulders and back). However, because of the contact nature of these sports, injuries can often occur.

## TRAMPOLINING

GOOD FOR:  FLEXIBILITY
TONING THE STOMACH AND LEGS
STRENGTHENING THE BACK
AEROBIC BENEFITS (IF MOVEMENTS ARE SUSTAINED FOR
15 MINUTES OR MORE)

Trampolining normally takes place at sports centres and is particularly popular with children and teenagers. Needless to say, it is important that it is properly supervised with people standing either side of the trampoline to prevent a fall. However, you can now buy a mini-trampoline or 'rebounder' for about £70 to use at home. These measure about 40 inches in diameter and nine inches in height, and although they are not nearly as bouncy as a big trampoline, they are, nevertheless, excellent for aerobic training and general toning. Like a proper trampoline, the 'give' of the surface means that the amount of stress placed on the joints is minimal.

You can do all sorts of movements on a rebounder including running, skipping, star-jumps and bunny hops, and if you combine this with large sweeping arm movements you will boost the aerobic effect.

Bouncing up and down on a rebounder is also good for relieving stress and can also be used for post-natal exercise and physiotherapy.

## WATERSKIING

GOOD FOR: STRENGTHENING THE ARMS, SHOULDERS, BACK AND LEGS

BALANCE

Waterskiing is a very exciting sport – providing you can brave the cold water in the UK! It is best experienced on calm inland waters. There are plenty of places where you can learn, but the most important things are to invest in a good wet suit and get good instruction. The teacher will usually demonstrate what you should do before you even get into the water, but the latest teaching method uses a 'boom', a metal pole extended from the side of the boat which beginners can cling on to while their instructor talks them through it. Once you have learnt how to get up on the boom, you can start using a rope extended from the back of the boat.

The hardest part about waterskiing is getting up out of the water. Once this is mastered, it is quite easy to keep your balance and skim along comfortably over the surface of the water. Mono-skiing (skiing on one ski) is more physically exhausting and requires very strong arms and legs, particularly when you slalom.

## WINDSURFING

GOOD FOR: STRENGTHENING THE ARMS, CHEST AND BACK

BALANCE

FLEXIBILITY OF THE BACK

TONING UP THE BOTTOM AND THIGHS (AT AN ADVANCED LEVEL)

Windsurfing is one of the most challenging and difficult sports to learn but one of the most captivating and rewarding once you are past the initial falling-into-the-water-all-the-time stage. You really do need good instruction and the Royal Yachting Association run an intensive beginners course (Level 1) that should give you enough knowledge and confidence to sail from A to B after a couple of days. Alternatively, you can learn a lot in a week's specialist holiday.

The attractions of this sport are similar to snow skiing – a tremendous feeling of freedom, adventure and tackling the elements. You don't actually need to be very strong or macho to learn how to do it – hoisting the sail out of the water is more about technique than muscle power. The sport is, however, excellent for conditioning the upper body. Once you get to the stage where you are sailing short boards in high winds, you will also start toning up your legs and bottom. It is also very mentally stimulating as you need your wits about you all the time in order to cope with changes in the wind direction.

I hope this part has given you some useful ideas about which sport you might like to take up. Don't be afraid to be a sporting butterfly for a while and change the sports you do until you find one that you really enjoy and which fits into your lifestyle without too many disruptions. Remember – all activity done properly is good for you and forms part of the *No Sweat Fitness* plan for a more active life.

# NO SWEAT RELAXATION

*No Sweat Fitness* is a balanced approach to health and fitness. And there is little point in devoting time and energy to getting your body in shape if your mind is in pieces. This chapter will help you evaluate just how stressful your life is, and give you lots of suggestions as to how to cope with this.

## HOW STRESSED ARE YOU?

Answer the following questions to see how you are currently coping with stress. Try to answer as spontaneously as possible and not to analyse the question too much. Follow your gut reaction!

1. How well do you sleep?

   A Very badly
   B Go to sleep easily but wake up a lot
   C Well, usually
   D Very well

2. Which of the following has happened to you during the last year?

   A A change of job
   B Divorce, or the end of a serious relationship
   C Moving house
   D The death of a spouse, partner or child
   E The death of a close relative or friend
   F Bankruptcy or redundancy
   G A baby
   H Marriage

3. At the end of the day, do you ever feel you need a drink to unwind?

   A Frequently
   B Sometimes
   C Never

4. Do you suffer from any of the following?

   A Headaches or migraines
   B Neck and shoulder pain
   C Poor circulation
   D Ulcers or problems with digestion
   E Fatigue
   F Poor skin
   G Palpitations
   H Constipation
   I Irritable bowel syndrome

5. How many days a week do you work?

   A Unemployed
   B Housewife or looking after young children
   C 5 days
   D 6 days
   E 7 days
   F 4 days
   G Less than 4 days

6. How do you currently feel about your job?

   A Very happy and satisfied
   B Fairly happy
   C Anxious about your prospects
   D Indifferent
   E Unhappy and dissatisfied

7. How do your currently feel about your relationship?

   A Very happy and secure
   B Happy
   C Insecure
   D Indifferent
   E Unhappy
   F Bored
   G Not in a relationship – and happy that I'm not
   H Not in a relationship – but wish that I was

8. Do you feel surrounded by people you can 'trust'?

   A Yes, lots of people I trust
   B Yes, one or two
   C No

9. How many times during the last year have you had a cold or flu?

   A More than 10 times
   B 6–10 times
   C 4–5 times
   D 2–3 times
   E Once
   F Never


10. How do you feel when you wake up in the morning?

    A Bright and breezy and ready for action
    B OK
    C Exhausted or depressed


11. Have you ever felt deeply depressed for no apparent reason?

    A Frequently
    B Once or twice
    C Never


12. When did you last have a holiday?

    A Within the last 6 months
    B 6–12 months ago
    C More than a year ago
    D More than two years ago
    E More than five years ago


13. Do you do any sort of relaxation technique (e.g. meditation, yoga, autogenic training, flotation)?

    A Yes
    B No


14. How often do you spend more than 15 minutes doing rhythmic aerobic exercise – like walking, jogging or dancing?

    A Twice a week or more
    B Once a week
    C Not very regularly
    D Never

15. How do you feel today?

    A Elated
    B Happy enough
    C Exhausted
    D Irritable
    E Depressed
    F Pressurised

16. Do you ever feel you have more than one thing on your mind?

    A Constantly
    B Only when I'm at work
    C Sometimes
    D Never

17. Do you have a good memory?

    A Yes
    B Fairly good
    C Not very good
    D Appalling

18. Do you ever feel you cannot cope?

    A Frequently
    B Occasionally
    C Never

19. How often are you late for appointments?

    A Frequently
    B Sometimes
    C Never

20. How would you describe your sex life?

    A Brilliant
    B Good
    C OK
    D Disappointing
    E Awful
    F What sex life? – and happy with it that way
    G What sex life? – but wish this would change

21. How do you feel about the future?

    A Optimistic
    B Uncertain
    C Never think about the future
    D Pessimistic

22. Do you sometimes feel you want to explode?

    A Yes, and I frequently do
    B Yes, and I sometimes do
    C Yes, but I am too scared of what I might say or do
    D No, I never feel angry

## ANSWERS

1. a = 4   b = 3   c = 1   d = 0
2. Score points for each tick: a = 3   b = 7   c = 4   d = 7
   e = 6   f = 6   g = 5   h = 4
3. a = 4   b = 2   c = 0
4. Score 2 points for each tick
5. a = 2   b = 2   c = 1   d = 3   e = 4   f = 0   g = 0
6. a = 0   b = 1   c = 3   d = 2   e = 4
7. a = 0   b = 0   c = 2   d = 2   e = 4   f = 1   g = 0
   h = 3
8. a = 0   b = 0   c = 4
9. a = 4   b = 3   c = 2   d = 1   e = 0   f = 0
10. a = 0   b = 1   c = 3
11. a = 5   b = 2   c = 0
12. a = 0   b = 1   c = 2   d = 3   e = 4
13. a = 0   b = 2
14. a = 0   b = 1   c = 2   d = 3
15. a = 0   b = 1   c = 2   d = 2   e = 3   f = 3
16. a = 4   b = 3   c = 2   d = 0
17. a = 0   b = 1   c = 2   d = 3
18. a = 4   b = 2   c = 0
19. a = 2   b = 1   c = 0
20. a = 0   b = 0   c = 1   d = 2   e = 4   f = 0   g = 2
21. a = 0   b = 1   c = 0   d = 3
22. a = 2   b = 0   c = 2   d = 2

# RESULTS

## OVER 65 POINTS

I am sure you are already aware that you are currently under a lot of stress. But the very fact that you are reading this book and answering this questionnaire means you are already doing something positive about it. First of all, don't be angry with yourself for being in this state and try to distance yourself from your problems for a while. Look at your answers above and say to yourself, 'I know I'm feeling angry/sad/depressed but I'm entitled to feel this way, so for the moment I'm just going to accept it.'

Don't try to blot your problems out – you must be aware of them but not too involved. Pretend you are a special 'stress reporter'. You 'observe' and 'report' that you are under stress but you don't judge it. You should never try to force yourself to 'relax' as this will only make you feel even more tense. The NO SWEAT STRESS POINT SYSTEM below will help you evaluate the stress in your life. Also look at your diet (turn to NO SWEAT NUTRITION) – you might well need to cut down on coffee, stimulants and anything that will make you more irritable and wound up. Finally, try to do as much walking and aerobic exercise as possible as this is an excellent way to unwind and elevate your mood.

## 40–64 POINTS

You are certainly suffering from stress but if you do something about it now you should be able to prevent it from going out of control. Do the NO SWEAT STRESS POINT SYSTEM. This will help you evaluate exactly what is causing you to be so wound up. Perhaps you are going through a major crisis at the moment, or maybe you are just reacting too strongly to minor problems. If the latter is the case, try to save your energy for the big stresses in life!

Check that you are eating a sensible diet (turn to NO SWEAT NUTRITION). Aerobic exercise is also very beneficial for dealing with stress (see AEROBIC FITNESS and THE WALKING PROGRAMME).

You are probably the sort of person who gets tense easily so it is important that you have a long-term de-stressing plan. We can usually cope with a large amount of stress in the short term but need to prevent a long-term build-up. If you lead a very busy life, try to organise a HOME RETREAT about once a month, and you may also be interested in taking up one of the relaxation methods described below.

## 16–39 POINTS

Although you are under stress at the moment, you seem to be coping fairly well. Try to pamper yourself as much as possible. If you can afford it, treat yourself to a weekly massage or a relaxing holiday, or alternatively, organise a HOME RETREAT (see below). Don't forget how beneficial aerobic exercise is for elevating your mood, and you may also be interested in taking up one of the relaxation methods described below.

## 0–16 POINTS

Congratulations! You are very calm and collected at the moment. Remember, however, that we need to *prevent* as well as cure the effects of stress, so now is a good time for you to lay down the foundations of a relaxed, healthy lifestyle. Check that you are eating a healthy diet (see NO SWEAT NUTRITION) and doing regular aerobic exercise, and perhaps consider taking up one of the relaxation methods described below.

## RELAXATION TIPS

1. Make sure you schedule time for relaxation as well as activity into your daily routine.
2. Our bodies are cyclical, which means they function best with regularity. Try to stick to a daily routine by eating, going to bed and getting up in the morning at similar times each day.
3. Make sure you have some time on your own each day. You may only need a few minutes just to lie down in a darkened room without any distractions.

4. Don't put yourself under pressure by taking on too many social engagements each week. If a friend rings up and asks you to go over for supper on your only free night that week, don't be afraid to say no if you would rather just stay at home in front of the TV.

5. Become a 'stress reporter'. Note how your body reacts under stress. Does it make you clench your teeth or jaws, bite your nails, tighten the muscles in your neck and shoulders, have sweaty palms or a tense nervous headache? Use the NO SWEAT STRESS POINTS SYSTEM below to monitor your reactions to stressful situations.

6. When you find yourself in a highly stressful situation, take a series of deep breaths and slowly count down from 30.

7. If you have a cat, stroke it! Research shows that stroking a cat, or a pet (or even your partner!) can lower your blood pressure. For the same reason, why not do a massage course? Giving a massage is just as relaxing as receiving one – so, if you learn how to massage, both you and your partner or friends will benefit.

8. Don't be afraid to tell people that you are suffering from stress. Acknowledging that you have a problem is halfway to solving it. Everybody is under stress to a certain degree so no one will think badly of you if you admit you are under a lot of pressure at the moment.

9. If you live in an urban area, try to get out to the countryside, seaside, or park at least once a week.

10. Don't bottle up your emotions. If somebody upsets you or makes you angry, tell them so there and then. Try to do this in a calm rational manner, again as if you were a 'stress reporter'.

11. Do some aerobic exercise. Research has shown that rhythmical continuous movements such as walking, cycling, jogging or dancing have an almost meditative effect and are a good way to elevate your mood. Try it for yourself – next time you come home from work feeling tense, go for a long, brisk walk.

12. Take up a relaxation technique such as meditation, yoga or autogenics (see below).

# THE NO SWEAT STRESS-POINT PLAN

It is impossible to eliminate stress totally from your life, but self-awareness is a great form of prevention. Use the charts below to record everyday events which are potentially stressful and mark them out of five as to how they make you feel. Also record any particular physical reaction you have (e.g. headache, tears, sweaty palms, trembling etc.), and pretend you are a journalist or 'stress reporter' who has been given an assignment about all this. Try to stay objective, keep a detached point of view and try not to judge your reactions. Re-read the charts in weeks to come, and you will probably look back and wonder why you reacted so strongly to certain events.

It does not matter what your total number of stress points is – this is not a test or competition – but it is important that you learn to award an appropriate number of points for any given situation. If you award five points, for example, when you find there is no milk in the fridge on Monday mornings, you are not going to be able to increase the score if you are suddenly faced with a big stressful event later in the week such as redundancy. Try to put stressful events into perspective . Don't waste time and energy worrying about the minor stresses in life – you need to keep some energy in reserve to cope with the big crises!

After a week or two you should find that you are awarding yourself more appropriate points and that you are learning to distinguish the minor from the major stresses in your life.

## STRESS POINTS

5  =  fuming/extremely distressed

4  =  angry/unhappy

3  =  annoyed/upset

2  =  irritated

1  =  mildly distressed

0  =  not stressed at all

## SAMPLE WEEK

| DAY | SITUATION | REACTION | SCORE |
| --- | --- | --- | --- |
| MON | Row with boss | Trembling | 4 |
| TUE | Car broke down | Swore a lot! | 3 |
| WED | Rude letter from bank! | Depression | 3 |
| THUR | Row with partner | Tears | 5 |
| FRI | Late for work | Panic | 2 |
| SAT | In-laws to stay | Boredom | 2 |
| SUN | Burnt lunch | Row with partner | 3 |

## WEEK 1

| DAY | SITUATION | REACTION | SCORE |
| --- | --- | --- | --- |
| MON | | | |
| TUE | | | |
| WED | | | |
| THUR | | | |
| FRI | | | |
| SAT | | | |
| SUN | | | |

## WEEK 2

| DAY | SITUATION | REACTION | SCORE |
| --- | --- | --- | --- |
| MON | | | |
| TUE | | | |
| WED | | | |
| THUR | | | |
| FRI | | | |
| SAT | | | |
| SUN | | | |

## WEEK 3

| DAY | SITUATION | REACTION | SCORE |
| --- | --- | --- | --- |
| MON | | | |
| TUE | | | |
| WED | | | |
| THUR | | | |
| FRI | | | |
| SAT | | | |
| SUN | | | |

## WEEK 4

| DAY | SITUATION | REACTION | SCORE |
|---|---|---|---|
| MON | | | |
| TUE | | | |
| WED | | | |
| THUR | | | |
| FRI | | | |
| SAT | | | |
| SUN | | | |

# THE NO SWEAT RELAXATION EXERCISE

Try the following exercise at the end of the day or after a work-out. It is a wonderful way to let your mind just relax and fill with a sense of calm. Imagine that your body is filled with a beautiful magical liquid that clears your body of stress and tension as it is drawn out of you.

## 114. NO SWEAT RELAXATION

Lie on your back with your head on a pillow, palms facing the ceiling and legs slightly apart. Close your eyes and spend a few seconds focusing on your breathing. Imagine that your stomach is a balloon that fills up with air as you breathe in and then slowly deflates as you breathe out. Do ten slow and controlled breaths like this.

Now imagine that your body is filled with a beautifully vibrant-coloured liquid. Choose your favourite colour, be it fuschia pink, emerald green or purple. This liquid possesses magical properties that will clean and empty your body of stress as it is drawn out of you.

Visualise that there is a stopper in the sole of each of your feet. There is a beautiful person who comes and pulls the stopper out of each foot so that the liquid can slowly drain out of your body, taking all the tension with it. Imagine the liquid emptying first from the top of your head, down past your temples and eyebrows, and past your nose, mouth and chin. Visualise each part of your body slowly being emptied of this liquid, moving down through your neck, shoulders, arms, wrists, hands, fingers, chest, stomach, hips, pelvic floor, bottom, legs, ankles and finally out through your feet.

To come out of the exercise, open your eyes, take a deep breath in, exhale and then stretch your limbs out as if you had just woken up from a long, peaceful slumber.

## DEALING WITH ANGER

It is important that we learn to let go of anger as anger turned inwards can lead to depression and despair. If you can't express your anger, you may be left with physical symptoms such as headaches, irritability, abdominal pain or anxiety. Indeed, in the long term, if you keep bottling up these emotions, you may eventually lose the ability to feel anger when you should.

First of all, you must dispel the myth that it is wrong to get angry. Women in particular are often afraid to let off steam but anger is an instinctive physical and emotional response to a potentially threatening situation, and used positively it can help to prevent stress.

Next time you find yourself in a stressful situation, try to verbalise your anger in a positive way. Again, act as a reporter on your own emotions. Don't judge them, just observe them. Tell the object of your anger how you feel but do not blame them for it as this is your emotional reaction not theirs.

Sometimes it can help if you can express your anger physically. For me, this involves screaming as loud as I can in the privacy of my car! You may find that stamping your feet, growling or beating a cushion has a similar effect.

The following exercise, derived from the ancient martial art aikido, is an effective way of releasing anger.

## 115. NO SWEAT ANGER RELEASE

Sit comfortably in a chair with both feet flat on the floor and a cushion on your lap. Bend your elbows so that your palms are facing you at shoulder-level. Let your fingers curl down slightly towards your palms – this should be a soft relaxed position. Now, without any emotion or aggression, start thwacking down on to the cushion with the backs of your hands. Make this a rhythmical movement and repeat it in a rather monotonous fashion like a child who is bored with banging a toy drum but keeps on going all the same! Try not to tense up or else you will get your adrenalin soaring too high again. As you thwack down on to the cushion, make a grunting or growling noise out loud. Keep repeating this until you feel tired or your anger has dissipated.

# HOME RETREAT

If you lead a highly stressed life, you occasionally need to take a total break and cut yourself off from the daily pressures. Some people like to take themselves off to a health farm, although personally I prefer to relax in the privacy of my own home. A home retreat will also, of course, save you a lot of money!

Here is a guideline to organising your own health and relaxation weekend.

1. Choose a weekend when you know you have nothing planned socially.

2. Make sure you have the house to yourself or that your partner has agreed to do it with you. If you have young children, arrange for someone to take them off your hands (and preferably out of the house!) for the weekend. Older children may like to join in, though.

3. Do your shopping on the Thursday night or Friday lunchtime, stocking up with all the food and drink you will need. Don't choose anything that will be complicated or time-consuming to prepare, and try to choose lots of raw healthy foods such as

vegetables, nuts, seeds and fruit, with mineral waters, herbal teas and vegetable or fruit juices to drink. Try to make sure that you do not buy anything that has been processed or refined (see pp207–10 for healthy eating guidelines) – you want to eat as little, and as pure food as possible this weekend.

Choose your weekend menu from the following:

## BREAKFAST

Porridge, cooked with soya or skimmed milk and a spoonful of honey;

*or* Sugar-free muesli, soaked overnight in soya or skimmed milk, served with nuts and fresh fruit;

*or* Natural yoghurt (Greek yoghurt is particularly delicious) with fresh fruit.

Drink herbal tea and a glass of fresh fruit juice.

## LUNCH

A large fresh salad with all your favourite vegetables (if you love asparagus, now is the time to splash out), slices of oranges, nuts and a squeeze of fresh lime juice.

A piece of fresh fruit – again, if you like exotic fruits such as mangos or papayas, now is the time to indulge yourself!

## SNACKS (whenever you feel peckish!)

Rice cakes (can be bought from most supermarkets and health food shops) – choose the unsalted variety

Fresh fruit

Sunflower seeds

Nuts (unsalted)

Raw vegetables, such as celery, carrots, radishes etc.

Mineral water

Vegetable juices

Herbal teas

DINNER

Jacket potato(es) served with fresh spinach and sprinkled with
    nutmeg;
*or* Brown rice served with steamed or stir-fry vegetables. Add Shoyu
    or Tamari sauce if you like.

You can swap around lunch and dinner if you wish. Remember –
only eat when you feel hungry, not just because you think you should.

4.  You should stock up on some beauty products, such as a body
    scrub, face peel and face mask, and also buy something to put in
    the bath, such as Epsom Salts (good for detoxifying), bubble bath
    or aromatherapy oils. If you are doing the retreat with your
    partner, treat each other to a massage and a facial – men enjoy
    facials just as much as women!

5.  Tell all your friends you are 'going away' that weekend. If possible,
    unplug the phone, so you cannot be disturbed. Hide all the
    clocks – you want to forget about time this weekend – and lock
    away the coffee and alcohol (avoid all stimulants and any biscuits,
    cakes, chocolates or fizzy drinks).

6.  Tidy up the house on Thursday night so that when you come
    home on Friday night it looks tidy and orderly. Buy yourself some
    fresh flowers as a special treat.

7.  FRIDAY NIGHT
    Prepare yourself a light healthy meal from the menu above and
    avoid the temptation to switch on the TV or stereo. You want
    the atmosphere to be as calm and peaceful as possible. Put candles
    in the bathroom, turn out the lights and have a long soak with
    your favourite oils or bubble bath. Afterwards wrap yourself up
    in warm fluffy towels, and if you feel sleepy go straight to bed.
    Otherwise, just lie down on the sofa and let your mind drift. If
    you are feeling very fidgety you can read a book but make sure it
    is nothing too technical or taxing. Remember – this is the weekend
    that you give both mind and body a rest.

8.  SATURDAY
    Allow yourself to be 'sinful' and get up when you wake up! You
    should have hidden the clocks away so it really does not matter

what the time is. Make yourself a healthy breakfast, then sit down and do the NO SWEAT RELAXATION EXERCISE above.

Spend the morning pampering yourself with a manicure or pedicure, or something self-indulgent that you do not usually have time to do. I like to take this opportunity to spend an hour giving my hair a special treatment with a wax conditioner.

Put a tracksuit or something comfy on and, after doing the NO SWEAT WARM-UP, either go out for a long brisk walk, a cycle ride or a jog. If you live in a city, try to go to the park or somewhere green.

When you come home, prepare and eat lunch. If you feel at all drowsy afterwards, go and have a sleep. Remember to take everything at your own pace this weekend.

Do the NO SWEAT HOME WORK-OUT in the afternoon. Try to incorporate as many stretches as possible, holding them for longer (up to 30 seconds) than usual. Afterwards, sit down in a comfy chair with a cup of herbal tea or glass of fruit juice. If possible, sit by a window so you can look out and let your mind drift.

If you are hungry, have your evening meal. Then take another long relaxing candlelit bath. This time give yourself a massage in the bath with a bar of soap! Use the edges to rub away any knotty bits or tension in the body. Start with small circular movements over the soles of the feet. Then work your way up your legs, over your arms and dig the soap into the knotty bits on your shoulders, neck and top of the chest. You will be surprised what a powerful massage tool a bar of soap can be! If you are spending the weekend with a partner, treat each other to this soap-bar massage.

After the bath, go to bed if you are tired. Otherwise, do the RELAXATION EXERCISE again and just sit quietly and read.

## 9. SUNDAY

Again allow yourself to be sinful and get up when you wake up! Have a leisurely breakfast, give yourself a body scrub and face mask. Put on a comfy tracksuit, do the NO SWEAT WARM-UP and go for an even longer walk, jog or cycle ride than yesterday. If you are hungry when you come home, have lunch.

Then do the RELAXATION EXERCISE and any other
beauty treatments you want to do. If you feel drowsy have a
sleep – otherwise, just read a book for escapism. Remember – no
TV or music!

Do THE HOME WORK-OUT, again concentrating on
doing long stretches. If you have any friends (not business
contacts) to write to, do so this afternoon. Make sure you keep
drinking lots of mineral water or herbal teas.

After dinner, have a final long relaxing bath. Do the
RELAXATION EXERCISE before you go to bed.

Remember to dig out your alarm clock and set it for the
next day, when you should wake up revitalised and bounding with
energy for the working week!

# RELAXATION METHODS

## AUTOGENIC TRAINING

GOOD FOR:  HIGHLY STRESSED BUSINESS-PEOPLE
                      ANYONE WHO WANTS TO LEARN TO RELAX WITHOUT
                      HAVING TO FOLLOW ANY SORT OF PHILOSOPHICAL
                      OR RELIGIOUS CULT
                      PEOPLE WHO WANT A DOWN-TO-EARTH LOGICAL
                      APPROACH TO RELAXATION

Autogenic training (AT) is a deep and powerful relaxation method
which was developed in the 1920s by the German doctor, Johannes
Schultz. The technique is very simple to learn and involves the daily
repetition of formulaic sentences such as 'My right arm is heavy' or
'My forehead is cool', and even if you don't actually believe in it and
are just practising the method, it can have such profound effects
on both mind and body that it needs to be done under medical
supervision.

Much research has been devoted to the effects of AT, and it
has been shown to be useful in treating a variety of stress-related
and medical complaints, including high blood pressure, arthritis,

insomnia, migraines, asthma, irritable bowel syndrome, skin disorders, anxiety and depression. In fact, I recently did a course in
AT, comprising eight weekly 'tutorials' costing £180 (which can be
claimed back on private medical insurance), and I can vouch for it's
being the most effective relaxation technique I have ever tried. Like
physical exercise, it has a cumulative effect – the more you practise,
the better the results. Initially, practice comes in the form of three
10–15 minute sessions per day which can be done anywhere – at
home, at the office, on the bus, train or even sitting on the loo! –
but after a couple of months you can carry on using AT for main-
tenance by just doing one 20–minute session or two shorter sessions
per day.

Everybody gains different things from AT – airline pilots use
it to help them recover from jet-lag while athletes use it to improve
their performance in competitions – but I find it helps me cope
better with the pressures of everyday life and put everything in a
clearer perspective. So, if you had a very high score in the stress
questionnaire at the beginning of this section, I definitely recommend
you consider it.


## FLOTATION TANKS

GOOD FOR: PEOPLE WHO CRAVE TOTAL PEACE AND QUIET
ANYONE WHO WANTS TO LOCK THEMSELVES AWAY FOR
AN HOUR
FANS OF THE FILM *Altered States*

Flotation tanks are light-proof, sound-insulated coffin-shaped cabins
that are filled with a highly concentrated solution of Epsom salts,
the idea being that you float on top of this saline solution (which is
kept at blood temperature) for about an hour in near-total sensory
deprivation.

Floating devotees claim that afterwards they feel calm, re-
energised and free of tension. As I suffer from mild claustrophobia,
this was not an ideal relaxation technique for me as I could not bear
it once the tank door was shut above me. However, you are allowed
to leave the tank door open and even the outside light on, although
this would seem to defeat the purpose of the exercise.

Some people absolutely love the sensation of floating – Peter Gabriel, for example, is said to write his songs this way – and it can be used to lower blood pressure, rebalance the metabolism, reduce pain (as it stimulates the body's production of beta endorphins, our natural pain killer) and accelerate the removal of lactic acid. As you are totally free from outside distractions, it also clears the mind and can therefore be used for learning, either by using audio cassettes or watching a video inside the tank.


## MASSAGE

GOOD FOR:  ANYONE WHO WANTS TO BE PAMPERED
           PEOPLE WHOSE TENSION MANIFESTS ITSELF IN PHYSICAL
           SENSATIONS E.G. KNOTTY SHOULDERS, PAINFUL
           NECK ETC.

Massage is one of the most pleasurable and effortless ways to relax. Many people deny themselves the pleasure of going for one as they think it is too self-indulgent, but it is not, however, just a superficial beauty treatment. A good massage can have profound effects on both mind and body, and can be particularly powerful for anyone who has been on their own for a long time and so denied the nurturing pleasure of human touch.

There are many different styles of massage. The most popular in the West is often called the 'Swedish' massage and is primarily used for physical relaxation, but like all types, this also improves the circulation and skin tone and can be stimulating as well as soothing.

Aromatherapy is a particularly powerful type of massage that uses essential oils extracted from flowers, leaves, bark and the roots of herbal plants. These oils are very quickly absorbed into the bloodstream and can be used to treat all sorts of ailments, including constipation, skin disorders, headaches, arthritis and sinusitis. On the other hand, Shiatsu is a Japanese style of massage that works on pressure points along 'meridians' which are supposed to influence the functions of various organs in the body. Shiatsu literally means 'finger pressure', although the practitioner may also use the pressure of his elbows, knees or even feet, and the massage is usually done with your clothes on without the use of oils or lotions so it is ideal for anyone who feels self-conscious about stripping off.

When going for a massage it is important to choose a good practitioner. Ask friends for recommendations and try to find someone that you have a rapport with.

## MEDITATION

GOOD FOR: PEOPLE WHO WANT TO DEVELOP THEIR POWERS OF
CONCENTRATION
THE SPIRITUALLY MINDED
ANYONE WHO IS INTERESTED IN LEARNING ABOUT
EASTERN PHILOSOPHY

Meditation is an ancient Eastern method of relaxing and revitalising the mind. Like autogenic training above, it has been proven to have many health benefits, including relief from insomnia, chronic headaches and hypertension. Many people teach themselves how to meditate from a book, although I personally found this too difficult.

One of the most popular types of meditation is called 'transcendental' meditation, brought to the West by Maharishi Makesh Yogi. A TM course lasts four days and teaches you how to meditate by silently repeating a mantra (or single word or secret to yourself), and, once you have mastered the technique, a 20–minute meditation session is said to be more refreshing than several hours' deep sleep.

## T'AI-CHI

GOOD FOR: PEOPLE WHO FIND IT IMPOSSIBLE TO SIT STILL AND
RELAX
PEOPLE WHO WANT TO LEARN A SELF-DEFENCE
METHOD AS WELL AS A PROFOUND FORM OF
RELAXATION
PEOPLE WITH BACK PROBLEMS

T'ai-chi is often described as 'meditation in motion', because this soft style of martial art, used by the Manchu Imperial Guard (the Chinese Emperor's personal guard), provides both physical and mental training. Its flowing, graceful movements are relaxing and meditative just to watch, but it also teaches you how to be 'rooted', so that, like the branches of a tree, your upper body will sway and move while the lower part of your body stays firmly positioned and undisturbed. As all the movements are done in an upright position, it is a good method for anyone with back problems.

Another benefit of T'ai-chi is that it can be done by all ages and is an excellent way to keep older people mobile. The exercises should be practised for about 15 minutes every day, and they teach you to turn your concentration inwards, strengthening the central nervous system, improving circulation and digestion and deepening your breathing. There is no need for any special clothing or equipment and you can do it anywhere, indoors or outside.

T'ai-chi is based on the Yin and Yang theory of opposites. For example, if one palm is facing upward, the other will face down, and force is *never* used against force. It is a very effective type of self-defence that shows you how to yield to brute strength, divert and then swiftly counter-attack, and this means that strength is not of paramount importance and women do have a chance against men. The aim of T'ai-chi is to achieve maximum effect with minimum effort.

## YOGA

GOOD FOR: PEOPLE WHO WANT TO COMBINE PHYSICAL AND
MENTAL TRAINING
PEOPLE WHO ENJOY THE SENSATION OF STRETCHING

Yoga is one of the most ancient forms of meditation, developed over 4,000 years ago in India. From the *No Sweat Fitness* point of view it is ideal, as it conditions both mind and body while increasing your flexibility, improving muscular tone and encouraging good breathing. It is also excellent for dealing with stress, working on the principle that a 'still body' leads to a 'still mind'. This is achieved through a series of postures or poses called 'asanas', many of which are given animal names such as the 'fish'.

This chapter should have given you lots of tips for leading a less stressful life. Don't expect instant results – like your body, your mind takes time to adjust to a healthier lifestyle – but keep looking at new ways to reduce stress in your life and you will soon start to feel the benefits. And when you become more relaxed, your physical energy will increase so that you will have more incentive to do all the other exercises in the book. Keep it up!

# NO SWEAT NUTRITION

Although this book is not claiming to be a diet book, nutrition is still an important part of the *No Sweat Fitness* plan as what you eat can have such a profound effect on your health and fitness. This chapter is not just for people who want to lose weight. A good diet will give you more energy and make you feel better whatever your shape or size.

## THROW AWAY YOUR SCALES

The first thing you should do when approaching *No Sweat Fitness* is throw away your bathroom scales – or at least store them at the back of a cupboard! How much you weigh is not relevant because it does not indicate what percentage of this weight is muscle and what percentage is fat. For example, when a friend of mine called John was 20, he weighed 13 stone and had a fine physique from running, playing rugby and weight-training. Ten years later, John stepped on the scales again and congratulated himself that he still weighed roughly the same even though he had no longer played any sport or exercise and was very unfit. What John did not take into account was that muscle weighs much more than fat so that his weight was actually very misleading. He had not exercised for many years so he had lost muscle and gained body fat. His weight was the same but he was actually a lot 'fatter'.

Many people make the mistake of assuming that if someone looks slim they must be fit and healthy. However, there are many thin people who are very unfit, with far too high a percentage of body fat, while there are many fat-looking people who are actually incredibly fit. Good nutrition and an active lifestyle is beneficial for *everybody*, whatever their shape or size. The only way to assess your body fat percentage accurately is to have it tested by a health professional with callipers or by hydrostatic weighing, but you can give yourself a rough assessment by seeing how many inches you can pinch in the test on p43.

# NUTRITIONAL AWARENESS

One of the first things you did in the *No Sweat Fitness* plan was to increase your body awareness. Similarly, if you are trying to lose body fat or improve your diet, you need to be aware of exactly *what* you are eating.

Unfortunately, it is very easy to trick yourself into thinking you are eating less than you are. Spend the next few days diligently recording every single thing that you eat or drink, including all the snacks that it is so easy just to forget about! For example, a day of a food diary may read as follows:

| BREAK-FAST | LUNCH | DINNER | SNACKS | DRINKS |
|---|---|---|---|---|
| **MONDAY** | | | | |
| coffee/milk/ | tomato soup | fish 'n' chips | apple | 1 can of coke |
| sugar | ham sandwich | tomato ketchup | chocolate | 1 orange-juice |
| croissant | white bread | peas | digestive | 3 pints of beer |
| butter/jam | mayonnaise | vanilla ice-cream | biscuits (2) | |
| | Kit-kat | chocolate sauce | peanuts | |
| | coffee/milk | coffee/milk | | |
| | sugar | sugar | | |

*REMEMBER! Write down everything that passes through your lips!*

| DAY | BREAKFAST | LUNCH | DINNER | SNACKS | DRINKS |
|-----|-----------|-------|--------|--------|--------|
| MON |  |  |  |  |  |
| TUE |  |  |  |  |  |
| WED |  |  |  |  |  |
| THUR |  |  |  |  |  |

FRI

_____

SAT

_____

SUN

_____

This food record will also be helpful when you start assessing the nutritional value of your daily food later in this chapter.

## NO MORE CALORIE COUNTING

If you've been on a diet, you've probably experienced the boring task of calorie counting. And it is easy to become obsessive about this and drive all your friends and family mad! Like standing on the bathroom scales, calorie counting, however, is a total waste of time as it does not tell you anything about the quality of what you eat. You may consume only 1,000 calories in a day, but where did these calories come from? Have you just snacked on chocolate and junk food? Are you actually eating a well-balanced diet?

Instead of worrying about how many calories you consume, you should start checking the nutritional value of the food you are eating. Below are some simple explanations about the sort of foods we need to eat and why.

## CARBOHYDRATES

Carbohydrates are the body's main source of energy, stored in the form of glycogen in the liver and in the muscles. Glycogen is the only food source for the entire nervous system, including the brain, and this is why low-carbohydrate diets make you feel so irritable and depressed – the brain is simply being starved of nourishment.

There are two types of carbohydrate – refined carbohydrates and complex carbohydrates. Refined carbohydrates are those found in foods such as biscuits, buns, cakes, white breads, sugar, honey and sweets, which have been removed from the plant that originally produced them. They are easily digested and make the blood sugar-levels rise very rapidly so that they give you an instant energy boost. This results in the pancreas (responsible for controlling blood sugar-levels) having to work extra hard by releasing lots of insulin to bring these levels rapidly down again. Your energy levels, therefore, flag too and you start craving more refined carbohydrates to pep you up again. It can quickly become a vicious circle. The more refined carbohydrates you eat, the more your energy levels surge up and down and the more you crave them. And if you keep repeating this pattern, you may eventually exhaust the pancreas and increase the risk of diabetes. And if that isn't enough, refined carbohydrate foods are also usually heavy in fats, calories and additives.

Therefore, from both a nutritional point of view and as a source of energy, complex carbohydrates are best for you. These are found in foods such as wholemeal bread, wholewheat pasta, potatoes, brown rice, vegetables, fruit (particularly bananas) and whole grains, and eating them, you quickly feel full up and satisfied. Instead of the instant energy buzz that you get from eating refined carbohydrates, your energy levels will increase slowly but steadily, thus giving you a lot more energy in the long-term and being much less stressful on your pancreas. Complex carbohydrates are also high in fibre which helps remove excess cholesterol from the body and keeps the digestive system healthy.

## FATS AND CHOLESTEROL

Fats are used to insulate the body and help absorb fat-soluble vitamins and protect all the body cells and internal organs. Fat is also used for energy when you are doing aerobic exercises.

There are two types of fat – unsaturated and saturated – and from a health point of view, it is the unsaturated fats which are better for you, as they can actually help reduce cholesterol in the body. Unsaturated fat is usually liquid at room temperature and found in olive oil, peanuts, avocados and fish. Saturated fats, on the other hand, are usually solid at room temperature and are saturated with hydrogen. They are found in animal products such as meat, butter, milk and cheese.

Cholesterol is only produced by humans and animals and is a hard fat-like chemical substance. There is not much cholesterol in most people's diet, but most cholesterol comes from saturated fat, which is converted into cholesterol in the liver. High cholesterol levels increase your risk of heart disease, so you should avoid eating too many saturated fats. As these are usually also high in calories, you need to reduce your intake of them if you are trying to lose weight.

Cholesterol is carried in the body by molecules made of protein and fat called lipoproteins. There are two types of lipoproteins – high density lipoproteins (HDL) and low-density lipoproteins (LDL). LDL are harmful as they release the cholesterol in the arteries and so increase the risk of coronary heart disease, the hardening of the arteries, high blood pressure and strokes. HDL, on the other hand, remove fats from the walls of arteries so reducing the risk of coronary disease. Saturated fats increase the level of the harmful LDL, while unsaturated fats decrease it.

The only way to find out if your cholesterol levels are high is to have a blood test. If you do not know your cholesterol levels, it is best to err on the side of caution and cut down on your intake of saturated fats such as fatty meats (liver, duck, goose, bacon, sausages and kidneys), butter, lard, full-fat milk, cream, biscuits and chocolate.

Although coconut and palm oil are not animal products, they too are high in saturated fats. Foods that can actually help lower your level of LDL include fish (particularly salmon, mackerel and herring), olive oil, groundnut oil and oat bran.

## PROTEIN

People in the West are much too obsessed about eating enough protein. It is no more important a part of your diet than carbohydrate or fat, but over here most people eat more than four times the recommended daily amount, an excess which can cause a lot of acidity, in the body. This in turn, can lead to osteoporosis (brittle bone disease), as calcium is taken from the bones to neutralise the acidity, and can also cause crystalisation in the joints and so lead to rheumatoid arthritis, quite apart from putting undue strain on the kidneys.

If you do eat too much protein it will actually be stored as fat, as the body regards any excess as toxic. This used to be a common mistake with bodybuilders as they thought they needed large quantities of protein in order to bulk up their muscles. Instead, they were, in fact, increasing their fat percentage, which usually resulted in an unwanted roll of flesh around the midriff.

Proteins are much more complex substances than carbohydrates or fats. They are built out of 22 different amino acids, ten of which are 'essential', as they cannot be made in the body. If you eat a steak, you are taking on a complete form of protein that has been made by the cow. Your body cannot use this and so has to break it back down into its component parts before making it into a protein it can use. This is why meat can be very hard to digest. However, if you eat food that contains the amino acids in their original form (e.g. in fruit, nuts and seeds etc.), your body can set about making its own protein straight away without having to break it down. Indeed, it is quite possible to get enough protein on a vegetarian (no fish or meat) and even a vegan (no animal or dairy products) diet.

## VITAMINS

Most people obtain sufficient amounts of vitamins in their daily diet. And if you are following the principles of balance in this chapter, you should not need to take any vitamin supplements. However, in some cases such as pregnancy and old age, some supplements may, in fact, be required.

# FOOD FOR HEALTH

*No Sweat Fitness* is all about being fit and healthy for the rest of your life. Crash diets are as useless as crash exercise plans. Sensible eating should be part of your everyday life and not something you do just for a few weeks to lose weight.

When you go on a diet, your body thinks it is being starved so it encourages you to slow down (i.e. your metabolic rate decreases). Your body also starts to store more fat as an extra reserve just in case you try to 'starve' it again, and this is why many dieters find that when they start eating normally again they put on so much weight that they are often heavier than before the diet began. This then becomes a vicious circle, as when they become overweight again they go on another diet.

## QUALITY NOT QUANTITY!

Instead of trying to cut down on the amount of food you eat, try to improve its quality. It is always much better to tot up a few more calories by eating good food rather than cutting back but eating poor quality food.

In a similar way to how you used your food diary, write down everything you eat and use the charts below to count up how many nutritional points you score in a week. Don't worry if you are eating some items from the MINUS sections. Remember – this is good nutrition for life and many people would be climbing up the wall if they thought they could never have a drink or a bar of chocolate again. Just try to improve your score over the next few weeks until most of the foods you are eating are in the PLUS categories, and then continue taking note of any changes in your energy levels or weight.

## PLUS TWO

Award yourself two points every time you have the following:

   Baked beans (no added sugar)
   Baked potato (eating the skin)
   Beans, peas and lentils (e.g. aduki beans, kidney beans, soya beans
      and chick peas)
   Dried fruit (preferably sun-dried)
   Fresh fish (wild trout, salmon, mackerel, fresh sardines, fresh tuna
      and cod are all excellent sources of essential fatty acids)
   Fresh raw fruit (bananas are a particularly good source of carbo-
      hydrates and energy)
   Fresh raw vegetables
   Homemade vegetable soup
   Nuts (preferably hazelnuts or walnuts – avoid salted nuts)
   Porridge
   Potatoes (boiled)
   Sea vegetables (e.g. arame, nori or wakame)
   Soya milk (delicious for making porridge with – but check that it
      does not have added sugar)
   Sunflower seeds (very nutritious for snacks)
   Tofu (curdled soya bean milk – high-protein, low-fat and low-
      calorie)
   Vegetables (preferably raw or steamed)
   Vegetable juices
   Wholegrain cereals (no added sugar)
   Wholemeal or brown bread
   Wholewheat pasta

## PLUS ONE

Award yourself one point when you have the following:

   Cheese (avoid full-fat cheese, choosing cottage cheese, ricotta
      cheese, low-fat cheddar, edam or gouda instead)
   Chicken (free-range without the skin: if you do eat chicken or red
      meat, try to buy free-range products, which means that the
      animals have been raised 'naturally')
   Eggs (free-range – if you suffer from high cholesterol levels, just
      eat the whites)
   Lean red meat (free range)
   Milk (semi-skimmed or skimmed)

Miso (made from fermented soya bean – excellent for making soup, but with quite a high salt content)

Olive oil (for salads and cooking)

Peanut butter

Rice cakes

Tamari (naturally femented soya sauce – excellent for cooking vegetables or fish)

Tuna fish

Turkey (free-range, without the skin)

Yoghurt (low-fat – add fresh fruit to natural yoghurt rather than buying fruit yoghurt)

## MINUS ONE

Deduct one point when you have the following:

Butter or margarine (if you do not suffer from high cholesterol levels, butter may be the better choice as it more 'natural')

Cheese (full-fat – but score plus points by choosing the low-fat varieties above)

Chips (try to choose chips that have been fried in fresh oil)

Coconut and palm oils (although these are vegetable oils, they are highly saturated)

Hamburgers

Honey (this is one of the most 'natural' refined carbohydrates)

Milk or cream (full-fat)

Pizzas (according to Tim Lobstein's book, *Fast Food Facts*, a cheese and tomato pizza is nutritionally one of the best 'fast foods' you can eat)

Tea (not as bad for you as coffee – but avoid tea that is 'well stewed')

## MINUS TWO

Deduct two points when you have the following:

Alcohol

Bacon and cured meats

Biscuits

Buns

Cakes

Chocolate

Coca Cola and fizzy drinks
Coffee
Doughnuts
Ketchup, pickles, relishes etc. (usually high in sugar or salt)
Mayonnaise
Salt
Sausages, sausage rolls, hot dogs and salamis
Sweets

| DAY | FOODS EATEN | POINTS | GENERAL WELL-BEING |
|-----|-------------|--------|--------------------|
| MON | 1 apple pie<br>1 slice brown bread<br>with butter + jam | | |
| TUE | | | |
| WED | | | |

THUR

_____

FRI

_____

SAT

_____

SUN

_____

WEEK 1:
TOTAL POINTS =

| DAY | FOODS EATEN | POINTS | GENERAL WELL-BEING |
|-----|-------------|--------|--------------------|
| MON |             |        |                    |
| TUE |             |        |                    |
| WED |             |        |                    |
| THUR |            |        |                    |

FRI

_____

SAT

_____

SUN

_____

WEEK 2:
TOTAL POINTS =

| DAY | FOODS EATEN | POINTS | GENERAL WELL-BEING |
|---|---|---|---|
| MON | | | |
| TUE | | | |
| WED | | | |
| THUR | | | |

FRI

_____

SAT

_____

SUN

_____

WEEK 3:
TOTAL POINTS =

| DAY | FOODS EATEN | POINTS | GENERAL WELL-BEING |
|-----|-------------|--------|--------------------|
| MON |             |        |                    |
| TUE |             |        |                    |
| WED |             |        |                    |
| THUR|             |        |                    |

FRI


SAT


SUN


WEEK 4:
TOTAL POINTS  =

# DIET TIPS

1. Eat plenty of complex carbohydrates (like wholemeal bread or pasta, brown rice, beans, pulses, potatoes). A low carbohydrate diet will make you feel irritable and depressed as carbohydrates are the main source of food for the brain.

2. Eat lots of fresh raw fruits and vegetables.

3. If you are lacking in energy, eat a banana!

4. Cut down on refined carbohydrates and fatty foods.

5. Olive oil is an excellent source of essential fatty acids, and can be heated to quite a high temperature without many changes taking place. Other oils become carcinogenic when heated above a certain temperature.

6. Never re-use the same oil to cook with as it will become more and more carcinogenic.

7. Go to the supermarket on a full stomach. When you are starving hungry you may not be such a good judge as to what foods you should buy!

8. Try to buy organic foods that have not been processed. Choose free-range meat whenever possible.

9. Don't drink while you are eating as this impairs digestion by diluting your gastric juices.

10. Think of your body as a high-performance racing car and give it the best fuel possible.

11. Try to eat small, regular meals, four to six times a day so as to avoid any binging attacks.

12. Keep some healthy snack foods in the fridge such as sticks of celery or carrots etc. and rice cakes – a healthy and filling nibble.